MW00614164

FOCUS GROUP
DISCUSSIONS

MONIQUE M. HENNINK

FOCUS GROUP DISCUSSIONS

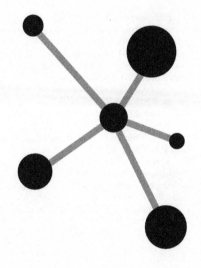

OXFORD
UNIVERSITY PRESS

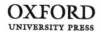

Oxford University Press is a department of the University of Oxford.
It furthers the University's objective of excellence in research, scholarship,
and education by publishing worldwide.

Oxford   New York
Auckland   Cape Town   Dar es Salaam   Hong Kong   Karachi
Kuala Lumpur   Madrid   Melbourne   Mexico City   Nairobi
New Delhi   Shanghai   Taipei   Toronto

With offices in
Argentina   Austria   Brazil   Chile   Czech Republic   France   Greece
Guatemala   Hungary   Italy   Japan   Poland   Portugal   Singapore
South Korea   Switzerland   Thailand   Turkey   Ukraine   Vietnam

Oxford is a registered trademark of Oxford University Press
in the UK and certain other countries.

Published in the United States of America by
Oxford University Press
198 Madison Avenue, New York, NY 10016

© Oxford University Press 2014

Library of Congress Cataloging-in-Publication Data
Hennink, Monique M.
Focus group discussions / Monique M. Hennink.
pages cm.—(Understanding qualitative research)
Includes bibliographical references and index.
ISBN 978–0–19–985616–9
1. Focus groups.   2. Qualitative research—Methodology.   I. Title.
H61.28.H45 2013
001.4'2—dc23   2013015633

CONTENTS

ACKNOWLEDGMENTS

I would like to thank Patricia Leavy for inviting me to contribute to this innovative book series, and for her feedback on the manuscript. I thank the many graduate students and workshop participants who over the years have provided stimulating discussions on qualitative research, which continues to encourage me to explore effective ways to explain theoretical and methodological concepts in qualitative research. I appreciate the Hubert Department of Global Health at Emory University for allowing me to take time to write this book during the summer of 2012. My sincere thanks to two graduate student reviewers, Lesley Watson (Emory University) and Jessie K. Finch (University of Arizona), who provided detailed review on earlier drafts of the manuscript. I greatly appreciate the assistance of Kate Cartwright (Emory University) with editorial tasks in the final stages of preparing the manuscript. I appreciate the generosity of those who prepared case studies to include in this book: Robbie Contino, Samantha Huffman, and the Leon Research Group.

Finally, I thank my friends and loving family for their continued support and encouragement, particularly my parents Albert and Celle.

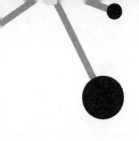

INTRODUCING FOCUS GROUP DISCUSSIONS

What is a Focus Group Discussion?

Focus group discussions fall within the qualitative research tradition. The name of the method defines its key characteristics, in that it involves a *focus* on specific issues, with a predetermined *group* of people, participating in an interactive *discussion*—thereby a focus group discussion. The method may be described as "an interactive discussion between six to eight pre-selected participants, led by a trained moderator and focussing on a specific set of issues. The aim of a focus group discussion is to gain a broad range of views on the research topic over a 60-90 minute period, and to create an environment where participants feel comfortable to express their views" (Hennink, Hutter, & Bailey, 2011, p. 136). The focus group method differs from other qualitative methods in its purpose, composition, and the group nature of data collection. Focus group discussions have several characteristics that distinguish the method, including the following:

- Focus groups typically consist of 6 to 8 participants, but can be anywhere between 5 and 10 depending on the purpose of the study.
- Participants are preselected and have similar backgrounds

or shared experiences related to the research issues (e.g., experience of an illness, multiple birth, divorce, and so forth).

- The discussion is focused on a specific topic or limited number of issues, to allow sufficient time to discuss each issue in detail.
- The aim is not to reach consensus on the issues discussed, but to uncover a range of perspectives and experiences.
- Discussion between participants is essential to gather the type of data unique to this method of data collection.
- The group is led by a trained moderator who facilitates the discussion to gain breadth and depth from participants' responses.
- Questions asked by the moderator are carefully designed to stimulate discussion, and moderators are trained to effectively probe group participants to identify a broad range of views.
- A permissive, non-threatening group environment is essential so that participants feel comfortable to share their views without the fear of judgment from others.

The essential purpose of focus group research is to identify a range of perspectives on a research topic, and to gain an understanding of the issues from the perspective of the participants themselves. The group environment enables a broad range of insights on the research issues to be gathered in a single sitting. Fern (1982) found that a single focus group discussion can generate about 70 percent of the same issues as a series of in-depth interviews with the same number of people. Therefore, focus group discussions can generate a wide range of data very quickly. Focus group discussions also enable participants to highlight issues of importance to them, thus giving more prominence to participants' perspectives on the issues discussed. A comfortable, non-threatening environment is important to provide participants with a "safe environment where they can share ideas, beliefs and attitudes in the company of people from the same socio-economic, ethnic, and gender backgrounds" (Madriz, 2003, p. 364).

Perhaps the most unique characteristic of focus group research is the interactive discussion through which data are generated, which leads to a different type of data not accessible through individual interviews. During the group discussion participants share their views, hear the views of others, and perhaps refine their own views in light of what they have heard. As the discussion proceeds participants begin to ask questions or clarifications of others in the group, which may trigger them to raise additional issues or share similar experiences, thus increasing the clarity, depth, and detail of the discussion. Morgan (1996, p. 139 cited in Hesse-Biber & Leavy, 2006, p. 200) states that "what makes the discussion in focus groups more than the sum of individual interviews is the fact that the participants query each other and explain themselves to each other...such interaction offers valuable data on the extent of consensus and diversity among participants." It is this synergistic nature of focus group discussions that leads to the unique type of data produced (Ritchie & Lewis, 2003). Indeed, "the hallmark of focus groups is the explicit use of the group interaction to produce data and insights that would be less accessible without the interaction found in a group" (Morgan, 1997, p. 2). Therefore, it is the group environment that brings out the variety of perspectives, but the interactive discussion that prompts rationalizations, explicit reasoning, and focused examples, thereby uncovering various facets and nuances of the issues that are simply not available by interviewing an individual participant.

In addition, focus group discussions are able to produce "collective naratives" on the research issues that go beyond individual perspectives to generate a group perspective on the issue discussed, which produces a different type and level of data from that gained in individual interviews. For example, in reporting results of a focus group study in Malawi, Mkandawire-Valhmu and Stevens (2010) describe a group narrative of "stigma and humiliation" experienced by women with HIV/AIDS, and a narrative of women's "powerlessness" to prevent infection because of gendered societal structures that lead to women's increased vulnerability to HIV. A well-conducted focus group discussion can therefore provide a unique type of data and perspective on the research issues.

In focus group discussions there is also a type of social moderation of the views expressed by group members, which provides an important quality check on the information provided. Patton (1990, pp. 335–336) states that focus group discussions can be a "highly efficient qualitative data-collection technique [which provide] some quality checks on data collection in that participants tend to provide checks and balances on each other that weed out false or extreme views." This type of social moderation results from the discussion component of the method and is therefore not evident in individual interviews.

Development of the Method

Focus group discussions are not new. The method has been documented as early as the 1920s and refined through the 1930s in social science research, but it gained most prominence throughout the 1950s as a tool for market research. Following its popularity in the 1950s the method largely fell out of use for several decades until it gained a resurgence in health and social science research in the 1980s (David & Sutton, 2004). Since then focus group discussions have become a core qualitative method in social science research and have been increasingly used across multiple academic disciplines.

Focus group discussions emerged because researchers wanted to explore alternative interviewing techniques that would overcome the limitations of traditional one-on-one interviews. In particular, they sought to ovecome the artificial nature of in-depth interviews with predetermined, closed-ended questioning, which could restrain participants responses or lead them to respond in a particular way. They also wanted to reduce the overall influence of an interviewer on a participant (Krueger & Casey, 2009; Hennink, 2007; Flick, 2002). These concerns were summed up by Rice in 1931, who wrote the following:

> A defect of the interview for the purposes of fact-finding in scientific research, then, is that the questioner takes the lead. That is, the subject plays a more or less passive role. Information or points of view of the highest value may not be disclosed because the direction given the interview by the questioner leads away from them. In short, data obtained from an interview are as likely to embody the preconceived ideas of the interviewer as the attitudes of the subject interviewed. (Rice, 1931, p. 561, cited in Krueger & Casey, 2009, p. 2)

These drawbacks of traditional interviewing led to the development of a new approach of non-directive interviewing, whereby the interviewer plays a minimal role and the dynamics of a group discussion are used to gather information (Krueger & Casey, 2009). The context of a group discussion is thought to create greater spontaneity in the contributions of participants because it replicates everyday social interactions more than a traditional interview. The function of nondirective interviewing is to shift the attention away from the dominance of an interviewer toward generating a discussion among participants. The discussion element of the method gives participants greater control of the issues raised in the dialogue, because they are essentially discussing the issues among themselves rather than directly with an interviewer. It is important to recognize that it is the creation of a group dynamic that enables spontaneous issues to arise from the discussion and for participants to highlight issues that are of importance to themselves. This element is less likely to occur in an interview that is more interviewer-directed. Ritchie and Lewis (2003, p. 171) state that, "in a sense, the group participants take over some of the 'interviewing' role, and the researcher is at times more in the position of listening in." However, they stress that this situation does not lessen the researcher's burden, because focus group discussions need to be carefully designed and managed for this to happen.

The principle of non-directive interviewing underlies the early development of focus group methodology in social science research. The approach of focus group discussions can be traced back to Emory Bogardus, a prominent American sociologist, who described using "group interviews" to develop social distance scales in 1926 (Wilkinson, 2004). During the 1940s, Paul Lazarfeld and Robert Merton at the Bureau of Applied Social Research at Columbia University used what they called "focused interviews" (Merton & Kendall, 1946) to examine peoples' reactions to propoganda and radio broadcasts during World War II (Barbour, 2007). They invited groups of individuals to listen and respond to radio programs designed to boost morale for US involvement in World War II. Initally participants were simply asked to push buttons to indicate whether they held positive or negative views of the programs. However, this method did not provide an understanding of why participants felt the way they did about specific programs. In subsequent work they used an alternative approach, which used an unstructured discussion format to provide a forum for participants to articulate their views and the reasoning behind their responses to the radio programs, allowing researchers to understand the complexity of participants' views in their own words. Merton (1987) noted that these group interviews produced a broader range of responses and elicited additional information than could be gained from individual interviews. This method was referred to as the "focused interview" (Merton & Kendall, 1946) in a paper published in the *American Journal of Sociology*, which became a landmark methodology paper at the time. Lazarfeld and Merton used focus groups as an exploratory qualitative research strategy, but one that was closely tied to improving their quantitative work (Madriz, 2003). Although Lazarfeld and Merton's new approach was significant, its impact was short lived, perhaps because of the prominent use of in-depth interviewing in the sociology discipline and the fact that sociologists rarely used group interviews in their research. During the 1950s the use of the "focused interview" faded and it was largely neglected in mainstream academic research for the following three decades.

During the 1950s focus group discussions were embraced in the commercial sector and used extensively by market researchers to identify consumer views on household products, develop brand identity, design product packaging, and gauge marketing strategies (Kroll, Barbour, & Harris, 2007; Bloor, Frankland, Thomas, & Robson, 2001). Since this time focus group research has become a mainstay in market research because it enables companies to stay in tune with consumers and provides highly valuable information from which to develop marketing strategies. Since market research is highly client focused, the approach to focus group discussions evolved from its original academic origins to suit commercial purposes. Therefore, market researchers often use specially designed facilities that allow commerical clients to observe participants discussing their product or innovation through one-way mirrors and discussions are frequently video recorded (Barbour, 2007). As a result of the popularity of focus groups in market research, specialist firms that provide services from recruiting participants in the client's market sector, providing venues with recording and viewing facilities, accessing professional moderators, and providing quick-time summaries of the group discussion to clients have mushroomed across US cities (Liamputtong, 2011; Conradson, 2005). Focus group discussions remain a core tool of market research firms to assess consumer views; however, their purpose and approach to focus group discussions differs from academic application of the method, as discussed later in this chapter.

In the early 1980s, focus group discussions gained a resurgence in academic research. Scholars initially adopted the market research approach to using focus groups, but realized that the commercial adaptations of the method were not well suited to academic research and they returned to the original intention of the method as devised by Merton and colleagues. However, researchers no longer saw the need to link focus group research to quantitative methods, as in Merton's work, but began to use focus group discussions as an independent method of enquiry to understand participants' perspectives on an issue per se. Focus group discussions now gained momentum in social science research. Knodel and colleagues were forerunners in using focus group discussions in social science research, applying the method to their work on understanding fertility and contraceptive behavior (Knodel, Havanon, & Pramualratana, 1984; Knodel, Chamratrithirong, & Debavala, 1987). Focus group research also became popular in the 1980s and 1990s during the emergence of the HIV/AIDS epidemic, to explore sexual behavior and sexual risk-taking in the context of HIV/AIDS (Liamputtong, 2011). The method also gained prominence with the publication of two special editions of academic journals highlighting research using focus group discussions (Carey, 1995; Knodel, 1995). During this time focus groups were also becoming familiar in the public sphere. In the United States focus group discussions were used during President Reagan's administration to identify public perceptions of relations between the United States and the Soviet Union (Stewart, Shamdasani, & Rook, 2007). In the United Kingdom focus groups were used by the newly elected Labour party in 1997 to gauge public perceptions of new government policies, in particular the introduction of fees for education. In the same year, focus groups were used to gauge public opinion on the role and image of the British royal family.

Focus group methodology has now become widely used across multiple disciplines, particularly in the health and social sciences, as evidenced by the increasing number of scientific articles and books on the method. For example, in the 5 years before 2011 there were almost 6,000 focus group studies published across the social sciences, with more than a quarter of these published in 2009 alone (Wilkinson, 2011, p. 168). Focus group discussions have wide application; they are used in health and behavioral research, evaluation of social programs, shaping of public policy, developing health promotion strategies, conducting needs assessments, and many more areas. Focus group discussions have become a well-established, valuable, and mainstream qualitative research method used across many fields of social research. However, the term "focus group" has become so well known outside research circles that many group discussions are incorrectly referred to as focus groups. This is perhaps most frequently seen in the news media whereby "town hall" style meetings or a media host engaging with a studio audience is referred to as a focus group, yet this type of exchange is not research and does not at all reflect the principles of the method.

New directions in focus group research continue to evolve. In recent years increased technology has seen the emergence of virtual focus groups using telephone and Internet facilities to conduct remote group discussions where participants do not actually meet face-to-face. Initially, virtual focus groups were used predominantly for market research purposes but they are being increasingly used in health, social science, and educational research (Liamputtong, 2011). These new applications of the method have practical appeal, in particular by increasing access to remote or dispersed study populations (Barbour, 2007; Bloor et al., 2001) and reducing the time and cost of conducting focus group research. The advantages and limitations of virtual focus groups are discussed next, and those of face-to-face focus groups are detailed in Chapter 2.

Two main types of virtual focus groups have emerged: via telephone and via the Internet. Studies may use both virtual and in-person focus groups to reach different types of participants in a study (Cooper, Jorgensen, & Merritt, 2003). Tele-conferencing technology has allowed focus groups to be conducted by telephone with participants in different geographic locations. In addition, video conferencing technology may be used so that participants are able to see each other during the discussion. In a telephone focus group (or telefocus group), the discussion is conducted in a similar format to a face-to-face discussion with participants joining the discussion remotely and a moderator posing questions and prompting discussion. A note-taker is usually present and the discussion may be recorded. Participants for telefocus groups are often recruited using comprehensive lists, such as physcician records or membership lists of professional associations (Cooper et al., 2003). Telefocus groups can be equally beneficial for a national study as for a study in a single location. For example, Hurworth (2004) conducted telephone focus groups in a study with elderly participants located in different suburbs of the city of Melbourne, Australia, whereas in another study with returned volunteers from the Overseas Services Bureau participants were dispersed across Australia.

Online focus groups are also becoming more popular and involve either synchronous (real-time) or asynchronous (not real-time) discussion. Synchronous discussions involve participants logging on at the same time to conduct a real-time discussion using an online chat room format (Bloor et al., 2001). These groups have some of the dynamic of a live discussion because they are conducted in real-time and led by a group moderator. However, participant contributions are typed rather than spoken, and this may make contributions shorter than in face-to-face groups. This format can be particularly useful for specific study populations, such as youth who are very comfortable using technology-based communications (e.g., chat rooms, instant messaging); those with mobility restrictions hampering their physical attendance at a face-to-face focus group; or those with concerns about attending a face-to-face group. For example, Fox, Morris, and Rumsey (2007) conducted synchronous online focus group discussions with young people who had concerns about their physical appearance because of having chronic skin conditions. Asynchronous discussions involve using a bulletin board format with participants logging in at different times to respond to the question posted (Ritchie & Lewis, 2003). Here, the focus group becomes a series of postings comprising a question from the moderator and contributions from participants. This format may be conducted over several days with participants agreeing to log on every day to make contributions. An advantage of the bulletin board format is that it allows a more reflective discussion, because participants have time to consider their perspective before posting a contribution (Krueger & Casey, 2009). This format may also be useful for participants in different time zones, or those who may be reluctant to participate in face-to-face discussions. In online focus groups, participant comments are typed and group members can see and respond to the comments made by others, thereby also creating an immediate written transcript of the discussion, which removes costly and time-consuming transcription.

Telephone and online focus groups share similar advantages over the face-to-face format. They can vastly extended the geographic reach of a focus group study by including particiants who are widely dispersed or in remote locations (Smith, Sullivan, & Baxter, 2009; Cooper et al., 2003). For example, telephone focus groups were used in Australia to access speech pathologists located in remote rural areas (Atherton, Bellis-Smith, Chichero, & Suter, 2007), and in the Unites States this format was used in a national study of physicians located across 17 states (Cooper et al., 2005). Virtual focus groups are also cost effective because of the elimination of transport and facility rental costs. Other advantages include greater comfort and convenience for participants who do not need to travel and can join the focus group from their own home or workplace (Smith et al., 2009). This can maximize participation and is advantageous for participants who are difficult to schedule, such as health professionals. An added advantage is the easier possibility to reconvene a virtual focus group if needed. There are also advantages with regards to participant contributions and group dynamics. Barbour (2007) suggests that in virtual focus groups a participant may be less likely to dominate a discussion compared with face-to-face groups, perhaps because of the absence of visual signifiers of status or body language that may lead some participants to dominate the discussion. Virtual groups also afford participants relative anonymity because participants cannot see each other, so it can be less intimidating for participants than a physical group, thereby potentially increasing participant contributions to the discussion (Krueger & Casey, 2009; Smith et al., 2009; Ross, Stroud, Rose, & Jorgensen, 2006). However, the advantage of anonymity may not be achieved in participant groups who are familar with one another through their professional or supportive networks (Smith et al., 2009).

There are also disadvantages to conducting virtual focus groups. The lack of visual contact means the moderator cannot observe nonverbal communication, such as facial expressions or body language, which may convey tacit information and visual clues that assist in managing a discussion and encouraging contributions.

This may make moderation more challenging and potentially lead to less detailed contributions from participants (Barbour, 2007). A moderator may need to compensate by identifying other strategies to develop rapport, show attention, and encourage participation that are not reliant on visual clues, such as altering their tone of voice, using reflective listening, or being attentive to participants who are not contributing to the discussion (Smith et al., 2009; Hurworth, 2004). Telephone focus groups are also shown to be smaller and shorter than the face-to-face format, thereby limiting the number of questions asked and the diversity of responses (Ross et al., 2006). Although anonimity of virtual groups may be an advantage, Smith et al. (2009) indicate that this can also result in inappropriate comments by participants, which can cause offense and disrupt group dynamics. This may be caused by the lack of social moderation in an online group compared with a face-to-face format. There is also the potential risk that participants in a virtual focus group will be interrupted, lack focus, or disengage with the discussion because they are able to conduct other activities simultaneously. Virtual focus groups also rely on participants' familiarity with technology (e.g., a conference call set-up or Internet technology) and risk being interrupted by technical difficulties. It can therefore be helpful to assign an assistant to bring participants online or into the conferrence call and to assist if they become disconnected.

Krueger and Casey (2009) state that virtual focus groups challenge the definition of a focus group by blurring the boundary between simple Internet chat rooms and focus group discussions. They offer the following advice to differentiate a focus group discussion:

> Internet groups become focus groups when the questions are focused, when participants are screened and invited to participate, when participants can freely and openly communicate without inhibitions or fears, when the moderator maintains control and moves the discussion in such a way so as to provide answers to the research question. (p. 182)

Virtual and face-to-face focus group discussions can play a role in qualitative research. Each approach provides a different contribution, and their strengths and limitations should be reviewed when selecting the most suitable format for a particular study.

Along these lines, Bloor et al. (2001, p. 75) state that "virtual focus groups are not the future of focus group research… However, virtual focus groups do offer a useful stablemate in the focus group tradition, and a worthwhile new tool for the social researcher." For a more detailed examination of the development and conduct of virtual focus group discussions, see Krueger and Casey (2009) and Liamputtong (2011).

Different Approaches to Focus Group Research

Focus group research has evolved over many decades and there now exist different applications of the method, each with variation in their purpose, procedure, and outcome. Considerable cross-fertilization has also occurred between these different applications of the method, such that it has become difficult to clearly define a pure approach to focus group research (Barbour, 2007). In addition, various disciplines have added their own specific adaptations to focus group discussions and advocate for their own context-specific approach to using the method. These various applications and adaptations can blur the boundaries between the different approaches and can make procedural advice across disciplines seem contradictory. Some of this confusion may be clarified by understanding the different goals and outcomes of each approach to focus group research. Four approaches to using focus group research are briefly summarized next by their use in academic research, market research, the nonprofit sector, and in community-based participatory approaches. These approaches are not exhaustive, but illustrative of different applications of the method for differing outcomes. The remainder of this book focuses on the academic application of the method. However, it is worthwhile to note that there exist alternative applications, to put the procedural advice offered in this book into a broader perspective.

The academic approach to focus group research is centred on the careful application of a research method, the generation of scientific data, and rigorous analysis of these data. Therefore, if done well, this approach can take considerable time. In academic research focus groups are often used to understand the context of people's lives or experiences, for example identifying the social or cultural norms of the marriage process or patients' experiences of seeking treatment for an illness. The method is used to identify diversity of experiences and perceptions and not to seek a consensus on the issues discussed. Focus groups may be used in evaluation research to understand why a service is not effective or to design health promotion strategies. The issues studied in focus group research may vary widely from public health, education, environmental concerns, public policy research, and many more. The academic approach typically involves conducting focus groups in community settings, such as the homes of study participants, community meeting halls, or in outdoor spaces. Participant recruitment is carefully planned and may involve segmenting the study population into different groups to avoid the creation of a hierarchy in group discussion, which may influence participant's contributions. Monetary incentives for participants are less common in academic research. Trained moderators use a carefully planned discussion guide to lead the discussion on specific topics of interest. The discussion is often recorded and later transcribed verbatim, which forms the scientific data that are analysed. Data analysis is a formal process, following accepted scientific protocol to code, categorize, and interpret the findings, and may use a textual data analysis program. Quotations from participants are often used in a research report to highlight issues raised. The research results are typically published in academic, technical, or policy reports. Overall the academic approach to using focus group discussions focuses on generating scientific data, follows a research process to ensure rigor and validity, and contributes to scientific knowledge.

The market research approach typically uses focus group discussions to gain consumer views on new products or marketing campaigns (Kroll et al., 2007; Bloor et al., 2001). This approach is heavily client oriented and pragmatic, with an end goal of making recommendations to a client on whether to launch a new product, how to improve the design of a product, or whether to adopt a particular marketing strategy. This approach is not concerned with the application of a methodology, but seeks to gain practical information and fast results for commerical decision-making. Focus groups for market research follow a more positivist tradition (Liamputtong, 2011), whereby questions are rigidly structured and highly controlled as in much quantitative research and seek to identify consensus among participants. Focus groups for market research are typically held in specially designed facilities with one-way mirrors to enable clients to observe the discussion. They use professional recruiting and screening strategies to gather participants from a specific market sector (sometimes calling on the same participants repeatedly) and employ professional moderators. Groups are often large in size (e.g., 10–15 people) and cash payments are given to participants. Given the specific goals of market research, there is often no need for a formal transcript of the group discussion, and if one is provided it is rarely subject to the detailed analysis that is expected of academic research (Barbour, 2007). The results are often generated within days of the group discussion and may comprise summary notes from a moderator, observations of those behind the one-way mirror, or a memory-based recall of the discussion points. The market research approach is unsuitable for academic research in which focus group discussions have a different purpose, procedural expectations, and outcome, therefore necessitating a different application of the method. However, the market research approach seems to dominate perceptions about how to conduct focus group discussions in academia, which can severly limit their use for academic purposes (Liamputtong, 2011; Kitzinger & Barbour, 1999; Morgan, 1993).

The public/non-profit approach generally uses focus group discussions for applied research. Information from focus groups is often used to design, improve, or evaluate a public service, such as a social program, public policy, or social marketing strategy. This approach is similar to that of market research, except the focus is changed from consumer products to social services or amenities. In this approach, focus groups tend to be smaller in size than for market research (e.g., 6–10 participants) to enable sufficient time for participants to share their views and concerns and to explore alternative opinions. Group discussions are generally held in the community and are often moderated by a member of the non-profit organization with skills in facilitation, interviewing, or evaluation. The approach to data analysis varies depending on the purpose of the research, and may involve a quick summary similar to that used in market research or a more detailed analysis, such as in the academic approach. Often the outcomes of this approach are presented as a summary of the key concerns or a ranking of the most important issues, with descriptive detail to convey the context of the issues.

The central tenet of the participatory approach, which emerged in the early 1990s, is to involve those who will use the results of focus group research (typically community members or groups) in the design and conduct of the group and the dissemination of the study results. This approach involves training, cooperation and willingness on behalf of the community to be involved in conducting focus groups, summarizing results, and making recommendations to the community. In the participatory approach, the purpose of focus groups is determined by community members themselves, because they directly use the outcomes. Using focus group discussions under the participatory approach may follow the broad procedures of the academic approach in terms of the conduct of the discussion and size of groups. The participatory approach is often used in community development research; community-needs assessment; and behavior change research, whereby the community itself has identified desired changes and wishes to use focus groups to discuss the barriers or strategies to achieving these changes (e.g., to promote healthy eating or improve hygiene behavior in the community). Using focus group discussions in the participatory approach has some challenges, such as the less consistent application of the method to each group discussion, the potentially variable skills of group moderators, and greater need for training of group moderators (Krueger & Casey, 2000). See Daley et al. (2010) for a description of using focus group discussions in community-based participatory research and the challenges of community participation.

When to Use Focus Group Discussions

Focus group discussions are a very flexible research method and therefore have a wide variety of applications. They are particularly effective for exploratory research, but are often mistakenly viewed as only applicable for this type of research. However, focus group discussions have much wider research applications, they can also be used for explanatory and evaluation research and can be a valuable component of mixed methods research designs. The results of focus group research have been applied widely to health, social science, and behavioral research; strategic planning; health promotion; policy development; program evaluation; and other areas of social science research. As with all methods of qualitative research, focus group discussions are not suitable for identifying the prevalence of an issue or for making broad population-level statements, which remains the domain of quantitative research. Various applications of focus group discussions are described in detail next. These are not exhaustive applications of the method or mutually exclusive, but provide examples of common ways to use focus group discussions. Focus group discussions are particularly suitable for the following research applications:

- **To explore** topics about which little is known or where the issues are unclear.
- **To explain** specific behaviors or beliefs and the circumstances in which they occur.
- **To evaluate** a service, program, or intervention and understand reasons for its sucess or failure.
- **To design** a survey or experimental study by identifying the issues, terminology, or components to include.
- **To gain diversity** of experiences and perspectives on the study topic.
- **To understand context,** culture, or social norms surrounding the research issues, because social moderation can distinguish typical from uncommon behavior.
- **To understand group processes** (i.e., decision-making) by observing how participants discuss an issue, influence each other, or decide on a strategy for action.

Exploratory Research

One of the most common applications of focus group discussions is for exploratory research. The group setting makes focus groups an ideal method to explore a topic about which little is known and to understand issues from the perspective of the study population. A group of participants can quickly provide a wide range of views on the research issues. The group environment is also highly suited to defining social norms or cultural practices, because the group discussion not only identifies normative behavior but the social moderation amongst group participants also distinguishes reporting of typical from atypical behaviors. Focus group discussions are particularly useful in the early stages of a study where they may be used to understand the research issues before developing the latter stages of the project. This approach is particularly valuable if the topic is complex or the issues are unclear at the outset. It may also uncover defining characteristics of the study population that can be incorporated into the study at a later stage, for example distinct subgroups of the study population from which separate data should be collected (Ritchie & Lewis, 2003). Figure 1.1 describes the use of focus group discussions in exploratory research to identify the beliefs and perceptions of diabetes among Bhutanese refugees in the United States. Focus group discussions identified a range of barriers to healthy eating and routine physical activity that reflected a participant's refugee experience, their migration to the United States, and deeply rooted cultural values and norms.

Focus group discussions are particularly effective for exploratory research in mixed methods studies. For example, focus groups can be used before quantitative work, such as a survey, to identify salient issues on which to develop survey questions, identify relevant response categories, and define concepts and terminology to include on the survey instrument. This approach can lead to the development of a more focused and relevant survey instrument, thereby increasing data validity. Focus groups can also be used to generate ideas for vignettes to use in a survey (Kitzinger, 2005). These applications of focus group discussion are particularly useful when there is insufficient information about the research topic or study participants to even begin to design a survey instrument. For example, O'Donnell, Lutfey, Marceau, and McKinlay (2007) used focus group discussions to improve the validity of a cross-national survey of physicians in the United Kingdom and United States. Focus groups were conducted among physicians in both countries to identify appropriate terminology to use on the survey, to test question comprehension, and to assess question relevance to each country. In addition, focus groups provided valuable information on administration of the survey, such as strategies to recruit physicians; acceptable levels of remuneration for survey participants (which differed in each country); and the type of organizational endorsement needed to encourage survey completion. Therefore, focus groups were used to strengthen the design of the survey and develop a more valid instrument by focusing on issues pertinent to the study population. The authors

Exploring Beliefs and Perceptions of Diabetes amongst Bhutanese Refugees

In 2006 the U.S. government agreed to resettle 60,000 Bhutanese refugees living in UN refugee camps in Nepal. Atlanta became one of the primary resettlements sites in the U.S. accepting over 5,500 of these refugees. This population has a high prevalence of chronic diseases, with 59% having diabetes, obesity, or hypertension, which prompted a community-based chronic disease prevention initiative. However, any initiative needed to be culturally tailored, understand the meaning attached to certain behaviors, and be congruent with community norms, understanding, and values. The purpose of this study was to explore the beliefs and perceptions of diabetes, hypertension, healthy eating and physical activity among the Bhutanese refugee community living in Atlanta to inform the development of future diabetes prevention initiatives.

This study was part of a larger community initiative utilizing the principles of Community Based Participatory Action Research (CBPAR), whereby community participation is sought in developing and implementing an initiative, the strengths and resources of the community are utilized, and the notion of equitable partnership development is built into the initiative to foster sustainability and ownership. Towards this end, a leadership committee was formed comprising nine Bhutanese community leaders, who informed the study design, implementation and interpretation of findings; in collaboration with researchers at Emory University in Atlanta. An exploratory research design using focus group discussions was used to identify the beliefs and perceptions of Bhutanese refugees on health and illness, and to explore the social, cultural, economic and historical influences on their beliefs. Four focus group discussions were conducted, which were stratified by two age groups (16-30 and above 40 years) in order to differentiate the health beliefs of younger migrants who have lived most of their lives in Nepalese refugee camps from older migrants who experienced traditional values of earlier years spent living in Bhutan. Separate group discussions were held with men and women. Focus group moderators were members of the Bhutanese community, trained by the research team, as per the CBPAR approach. Four key informant interviews were also conducted to provide context to issues raised in focus group discussions.

Results showed that both older and younger participants had a basic understanding of healthy eating and physical activity that are congruent with Western biomedicine. However, they described a range of barriers to healthy eating and routine physical activity that reflect their prolonged refugee state, their migration experience to the US, and deeply rooted cultural values and norms. Focus group participants explained that the main barrier to healthy eating was the desire to maintain traditional eating habits, which included large quantities of rice with each meal and using generous amounts of salt, sugar, and butter in food preparation.

Figure 1.1. Use of focus group discussions for exploratory research.

Older participants stated that the refugee experience exacerbated their desire to maintain familiar traditional habits while displaced and in difficult circumstances. They also explained how social pressure and collectivist values led them to conform to traditional food preparation, as food is prepared collectively for the extended family therefore altering personal eating habits is difficult. Younger participants described that in refugee camps unhealthy food was visible but not affordable and food rations gave little variety in their diet. However, when they were in the U.S. a large variety of unhealthy food was affordable so they now consumed excessive amounts of 'junk' food, (high in fat and sugar), which they were previously denied. One of the main barriers to physical activity was lack of time, as in the U.S. refugees hold jobs with long and non-traditional working hours, including nights, evenings, and weekends, leaving no time to exercise. In this study, using focus group discussions enabled an exploration of the underlying social, cultural, and migration influences on refugees diet and physical activity, which could later be used to design specific health interventions for this study population.

R. Contino (2012)

Figure 1.1. (Continued)

also report that conducting focus group discussions before the survey reduced the overall cost of the study by eliminating unusable survey questions; shortening the survey, which enhanced participation; and avoiding wasted time in analyzing unusable survey data.

Focus group discussions can also provide valuable information when designing a social product (e.g., health education materials) or intervention (e.g., new policy or program), to identify the words, images, and slogans to include (and exclude) to appeal to the target population. Focus group discussion can also be used before conducting in-depth interviews to explore the broad issues to include in the in-depth interviews where they can be explored in greater depth. Alternatively, focus group discussions may be conducted after in-depth interviews to discuss the issues, debate strategies, or confirm experiences heard in the interviews more broadly.

Explanatory Research

Focus group discussions are an effective tool for explanatory research. One of the primary reasons to conduct qualitative research is often to explain why certain behaviors or phenomenon occur. Focus group discussions provide a unique forum for participants to not only describe certain beliefs, behaviors, or attitudes but also to identify the underlying context in which they occur, enabling an explanation of why certain phenomena persist. For example, one may wish to explain why people continue to text message while driving despite the risks and warning campaigns against it or why some people believe strongly that free health services are of inferior quality to those that charge a fee. Focus group discussions provide an ideal forum for participants to discuss and debate these issues. Furthermore, several focus group discussions may be conducted with different sub-groups of the study population, thereby allowing comparison among groups that can further contribute to explaining phenomenon. For example, the reasons why young men text message while driving may be different from reasons given by young women, thereby providing important nuance to the explanation of the phenomenon. Figure 1.2 describes how focus group discussions were used to explain why labor migrants to Kazakhstan were vulnerable to developing tuberculosis. Results highlighted three underlying structural contexts that increased a migrant's risk for contracting tuberculosis and reduced their likelihood of seeking treatment.

Explaining Labor Migrants' Vulnerability to Tuberculosis

Kazakhstan has become an important destination for undocumented seasonal labor migration from Uzbekistan. Due to the high incidence of tuberculosis (TB), TB treatment is provided free of charge in Kazakhstan, but migrants rarely access this free treatment or health services in general. This study sought to explain the mechanisms that impede migrant workers' access to free TB treatment in Kazakhstan.

Twelve focus group discussions were held with Uzbek labor migrants, in addition to in-depth interviews with TB patients and health workers. The study was conducted in the main sending and receiving areas for migrants in both Uzbekistan and Kazakhstan. Ten focus group discussions were held with male labor migrants employed in construction, trade and restaurant work, and two with female labor migrants employed in cotton picking and service industries. Focus group participants were recruited at their places of employment, including markets, construction sites and cotton fields. Group

---

Figure 1.2. Use of focus group discussions for explanatory research. Reproduced with permission from Huffman, S., Veen, J., Hennink, M., and McFarland D. "Exploitation, Vulnerability to Tuberculosis and Access to Treatment among Uzbek Labor Migrants in Kazakhstan," 2012, *Social Science and Medicine, 74*, pp. 864–872.

discussions focused on migrants' living and working conditions, awareness of TB, experiences of illness, health seeking behavior and access to health care. In-depth interviews provided more personal narratives of TB patients' treatment and care, and health providers' experiences and attitudes towards treating migrants. Group discussions were conducted in Russian, Uzbek, and Karakalpak. Data were analyzed using the grounded theory approach to develop a conceptual model (see figure below) showing the structural influences on migrants' vulnerability to TB and barriers to seeking treatment.

Focus group discussions were valuable in identifying three structural contexts which shape migrants' daily lives – their legal, employment, and health care contexts. These contexts overlapped to create a vulnerable environment, whereby migrants were both at increased risk of contracting TB and were less likely to seek treatment, thereby increasing the severity of the disease. For example, migrants' employment context placed them in casual labor with no formal registration where they were overworked and provided with poor housing conditions. This overlapped with their legal context, where they experienced police raids, leading them to hide from police and formal services fearing harassment and deportation. This situation in turn influenced their health care context, as they were reluctant to access formal health services, fearing bribes and poor attitudes towards migrants. These three contexts together increased migrants' vulnerability to TB and discouraged treatment seeking, albeit free. The in-depth interviews validated these structural barriers and provided more personal narratives of health seeking, providing greater detail to link the three structural contexts.

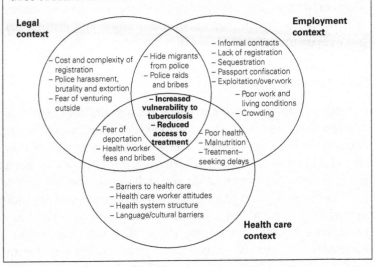

Figure 1.2. (Continued)

Focus group discussions can also be used as an explanatory tool in mixed methods research designs. In this case, focus groups are conducted as a successor to quantitative work to explain, clarify, or provide contextual insight to the findings of the quantitative research. This explanatory capacity of focus group research is perhaps the most underused (Hennink, 2007). Quantitative research often identifies strong relationships between variables but cannot provide explanations about why these linkages exist (Green & Thorogood, 2004). Survey findings may also reveal confusing or seemingly contradictory results. Focus group discussions may therefore be used after quantitative research to uncover contextual information and provide examples, enabling a fuller understanding of the quantitative findings. Focus groups can also be used to "tease out the reasons for surprising or anomalous findings and to explain the occurrence of 'outliers' identified—but not explained— by quantitative approaches" (Kitzinger, 2005, p. 59). The contributions of focus group data enable more powerful and nuanced explanations of the quantitative findings and may challenge how quantitative data are typically interpreted (Liamputtong, 2011). Furthermore, focus group discussions can be used subsequent to a survey to explore specific sub-groups of the study population, which exist in insufficient numbers in the survey data for statistical analysis but which may uncover important and distinct perspectives on the research issues (Ritchie & Lewis, 2003).

Evaluation Research

Focus group discussions are an effective diagnostic tool for evaluation research, to examine the effectiveness of a service or program. Focus groups can uncover the strengths and weaknesses of a service and identify how it can be delivered more effectively. Focus group discussions in evaluation research enable you not only to identify the drawbacks of a service or program, but perhaps more importantly, to understand why these deficiencies exist and how to improve specific components of a service. This information is invaluable for program evaluation and planning. For example, the Civil Aviation Authority in the United Kingdom used focus group discussions to identify the experiences of aircraft noise among residents near a major international airport. The results were used to evaluate the potential impact of changing the current no-fly policy between midnight and 6 a.m. (Diamond et al., 2000). Similarly, the Government of Malawi commissioned focus group research to assess the effect on poor communities of introducing a fee for family planning services (Hennink & Madise, 2005). Focus group discussions were also used to examine how media messages about HIV/AIDS during the 1990s were processed by the community and how they influenced peoples' perceptions of AIDS (Kitzinger, 1994 cited in Green & Thorogood, 2004). Figure 1.3 describes how focus group research was used to evaluate a health directory developed for the Latino population, and provided valuable

---

Evaluating Health Materials for the Latino Community

The Latin American population in the USA has a low use of health care services, partly due to the lack of culturally appropriate information on the health services available. The purpose of this study was to develop and evaluate a comprehensive resource guide of Spanish-speaking health services in the city of Atlanta, with an emphasis on free or low cost services, given the low income of the target population.

An initial resource guide was developed by conducting a survey of 1,000 health providers in the city to identify services offered; 210 of those that responded met the inclusion criteria for the resource guide by having Spanish-speaking staff or access to interpretation services. The resource guide was developed in Spanish and the format was based on similar guides used in other cities, which included a brief description of each health provider and a table of their services and characteristics. The cover page of the guide was particularly important as it needed to appeal to the Latino community. It was initially developed using known themes for marketing to the Latino population, such as images expressing emotions and family interaction.

Focus group discussions and in-depth interviews were conducted to evaluate the usability and appropriateness of the resource guide amongst the Latino population. Focus group discussions were held with Latina health advocates (promotoras) who have frequent interaction with the Latino population and knowledge of their health issues. A trained moderator led the group discussions on the appeal of the cover design, usability of the format and relevance of information provided. Strategies for publicizing and distributing the resource guide were also discussed.

Results of the focus group discussions identified important refinements to the resource guide to improve its appropriateness for the Latino population. Focus group participants highlighted that the cover page needed to include bright colors, images of Latino people with similar skin tones to themselves, reflect their social status and be dressed in clothing styles reflective of their

Figure 1.3. Use of focus group discussions for evaluation research.

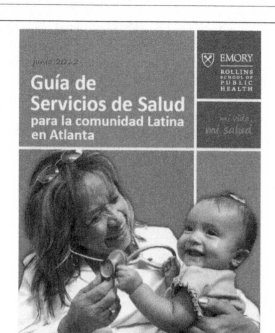

community. The health terminology needed to be simplified, for example 'substance abuse' was replaced with 'addiction to drugs and alcohol' and the phrase 'proof of residence' caused concern as it was confused with legal status and was rephrased. Given variable literacy amongst this population, additional visual aids were recommended (e.g. illustrations, maps). In-depth interviews were also held with Latino community members who identified the same issues for refining the resource guide. Findings were used to redesign the resource guide and the cover page (shown above).

Further focus group discussions will be conducted to evaluate the improved guide amongst health providers (who may use the guide for referral), and members of the Latino community.

Francisco S. Palomeque, Gaelle Gourmelon & Juan Leon
from the **Leon Research Group, Emory University**

Figure 1.3. (Continued)

information on the design of the directory, including the most appropriate images, words, and colors to use that would appeal to the target population. Evaluation research may also combine focus group discussions with observation approaches. For example, focus group participants may report issues with privacy in a clinic, whereas observation may reveal that the consultation rooms are separated only by curtains providing no audio privacy or that glass partitions in a registration area provide no visual privacy. Using a combination of methods provides different perspectives on the study issues.

Mixed Methods Research

Focus group discussions can be used as an independent research method or they can be used in mixed methods research as described previously. For example, focus groups can be conducted before quantitative research (e.g., in exploratory research) or subsequent to quantitative research (e.g., in explanatory research). However, the use of focus group discussions in mixed methods research is not only limited to their use before or after quantitative research. They can also be used in parallel to quantitative methods or as part of a broader research approach, such as ethnography or community-based participatory action research, where a range of research methods are used, each with a different purpose.

The goal of using qualitative and quantitative methods in parallel is to gain a broader understanding of the research issue that no single method alone can provide, so each approach illuminates different aspects of a research problem. For example, quantitative methods can measure the research problem, whereas focus group discussions can explore more complex aspects of the research issue that are difficult to include on a survey instrument, thereby contributing a more contextual understanding of the issues. For example, Lam, Fielding, Johnson, Tin, and Leung (2004) used focus group discussions in parallel to a randomized controlled trial to identify barriers to practicing evidence-based medicine among medical undergraduates. A longitudinal research design was used whereby focus groups were conducted at three time points, before, during, and after the trial intervention to identify students' changing attitudes toward adopting evidence-based medicine. The use of focus group discussions in mixed methods research is seen as increasingly valuable in social science research. For a more detailed discussion of combining focus group discussions with quantitative research, see Green and Thorogood (2004), Ritchie and Lewis (2003), and Tashakkori and Teddlie (1998).

When Not to Use Focus Group Discussions

Sometimes focus group discussions are not the most appropriate method to use, and can lead to poor quality data as a result. Most situations where focus groups are not ideal result from the group nature of data collection, which influences the topics that can be discussed or the type of data that can be collected.

Focus group discussions are not suitable when aiming specifically to collect personal experiences from participants. It is inappropriate to ask focus group participants to share personal experiences in a group setting, because of the lack of confidentiality. Questions on a focus group discussion guide are therefore often phrased more broadly than in an in-depth interview guide. Although some focus group participants inevitably share their personal experience despite the group setting, they do so of their own volition rather than as an expectation of the study design.

Focus group discussions are not useful for eliciting individual narratives from each participant. This is primarily because participants may be reluctant to share their individual story with a group of people but also because of the logistics of allowing each participant to provide a personal narrative about each discussion topic. There is insufficient time in a focus group for this to happen and it is likely that individual narratives will be fragmented, incomplete, and confused as others contribute, interrupt, or question the speaker. This is particularly true if attempting to seek process information from each individual in a group discussion (e.g., their process of marriage, migration, illness, and so forth). Barbour (2007) states that this may be achieved in smaller focus group discussions, however, if narrative data are desired, an in-depth interview is often a more suitable format because there is more time for a participant to describe their personal story in detail and the data may be collected in a more logical and sequential way. In addition, focus groups should not be seen as equivalent to an individual interview with six to eight participants. It is important to remember that data from a focus group discussion are the product of group interaction, discussion, and debate, which influences the contributions of individual participants. Focus group discussions may therefore not fully represent the perspective of individual participants in the same way as an individual interview.

It is often said that focus group discussions are not suitable for sensitive topics. However, it is not the topic per se but rather the focus of the topic that influences its suitability for a focus group discussion. For many years focus group discussions have been a core method used in research on sexual behavior, contraceptive use, abortion, terminal illness, suicide, mental illness, palliative care, and other clearly sensitive topics (Barbour, 2007). Therefore, focus group discussions can be used to discuss sensitive topics; however, the group discussion is not being used to ask about participants' personal experiences on these topics, instead focusing on broader perspectives. For example, a focus group discussion on the topic of sexual risk behavior may ask participants to describe situations where they believe unprotected sex occurs among people of their age, what can be done to encourage safer sex, and the best channels to provide safer sex messages. Although the topic of sexual behavior may be considered sensitive, the focus of the questions is broad and does not require participants to explicitly share their personal experiences of unsafe sex. Conversely, it may be too confronting to ask participants specifically about their own experiences of unsafe sex in a group setting. Similarly, a study on induced abortion may use focus group discussions to identify community attitudes on the topic, and then use in-depth interviews to discuss an individual's personal experience of having an abortion. Therefore, the specific focus of the topic needs to be considered in deciding whether or not it is too sensitive for a group discussion, rather than ruling out entire topics per se. In other situations, the group setting may offer a supportive environment in which to discuss sensitive topics. For example, it may be appropriate to use focus group discussions in a study on suicide if participants are selected because they have considered suicide. In this situation, the group enviroment may offer solidarity in discussing this issue, especially if the focus group comprises an existing support group where participants are already familiar with one another. In summary, it is not sufficient to identify that a topic per se is too sensitive for a group discussion without considering the focus of the topic and the type of group participants.

Focus group discussions are designed to seek diversity in perspectives and may be less suited to reaching a consensus on the research issues. Lastly, focus group discussions aim to provide a comfortable environment where participants can share their views openly. Thus, it may not be fruitful to include participants with highly confrontational views in a single focus group discussion (e.g., activists from pro-gun and anti-gun standpoints), rather hold separate groups for each.

Focus Group Discussion or In-Depth Interview?

It may be unclear whether to use focus group discussions or in-depth interviews for a particular study. It should not be assumed that the methods are simply interchangable. There are no definitive rules on which method to select for a given type of project, because this largely depends on the nature of the research topic, purpose of the study, type of data sought, and the characteristics of participants. However, some general guidance can be given on which method to select. The following broad distinctions can be made about when to use focus group discussions versus in-depth interviews (Box 1.1).

When selecting between focus group discussions and in-depth interviews, consider the benefits and drawbacks of the group environment of a focus group discussion. With a group of participants, a broad range of views and perspectives can be captured in a single session, participants can discuss and debate issues thereby uncovering justifications and reasoning for different perspectives, and

---

Box 1.1 Focus Group Discussions Versus In-Depth Interviews

....

Use Focus Group Discussions	Use In-Depth Interviews
To capture a range of views and experiences	To seek individual perspectives
To discuss or explain issues	To identify individual narratives
To explore new issues	To seek personal and sensitive information
To identify social and community norms	To collect detailed, in-depth information
To seek broad community-level information	To describe complex issues or processes
To observe group interaction	For geographically dispersed participants

participants can also collectively explain phenomenon providing a range of influences and nuances around an issue. Furthermore, the group environment provides an effective forum for exploring new topics, generating community-level information, and identifying social and community norms. If these outcomes are desired, then focus group discussions are ideal. However, the group environment also has drawbacks. The group setting is less confidential, a group of people inevitably generates less detailed information, and some issues may not be suitable to discuss in a group.

In-depth interviews offer a different dynamic to focus group discussions, with the entire interview focused on a single participant. This offers the opportunity to explore issues in greater depth and to collect personal narratives and individual experiences from participants. An interviewer can probe a participant for greater depth, examples, and clarifications in a way that is more challenging in a group setting. In-depth interviews can explore complex topics and process information much more effectively than in a group discussion (e.g., describing the nuances of household decision-making or personal experiences during the process of migration). The increased confidentiality of an in-depth interview allows for more personal information to be described than can be included in a group discussion. If these outcomes mirror the goals of a research project then in-depth interviews are more suitable than focus group discussions. However, the individual focus of data collection does not allow for discussion of issues or any social moderation of views and the interviewer cannot immediately cross-check information provided by a participant in the same way as in a group discussion. Overall, the benefits and drawbacks of each method of data collection need to be considered in relation to the goals of a specific research project to select the most approporate method of data collection.

Strengths and Limitations of Focus Group Discussions

Focus group discussions have many advantages, which are summarized in Figure 1.4. First, the group setting reflects people's natural tendency for social interaction to discuss issues in a group. Some participants find this an enjoyable experience, which influences the quality of the data collected.

Strengths	Limitations
Social setting: Replicates social interaction Comfortable environment	**Skills required:** Requires a skilled moderator Less controlled environment Need comfortable environment
Flexiblity: Useful for exploratory, explanatory, and evaluative research Suitable for mixed method research Use group activities to prompt discussion	**Group dynamics:** Some participants may dominate Some participant may not contribute Influence of social pressure Hierarchies may develop Non-confidential setting
Group environment: Generates large volume of data Elicits a range of views Limited researcher influence Participants identify issues Identifies new issues Issues debated and justified Social moderation of issues	**Data and analysis:** Few issues discussed Responses not independent Issues can lack depth Large volume of data Data analysis time consuming and costly

Figure 1.4. Strengths and limitations of focus group discussions. Adapted and reproduced with permission from Hennink, M., 2007, "*International focus group research: A handbook for the health and social sciences,*" Cambridge: Cambridge University Press, p. 7.

A second advantage is the flexibility of the method, which can be applied to a variety of research needs depending on the level of structure used. For example, focus groups can be relatively unstructured where the research is exploratory and the issues unknown. Focus groups can also be more structured for explanatory or evaluative research where the purpose is more focused. The flexible application of the method also makes it well suited for use in mixed methods research. The group format is also very amenable for using activities to prompt a discussion, and can also contribute to developing group rapport.

Perhaps the greatest strength of the method comes from the group environment in which data are collected. A 1-hour focus group discussion can generate a large volume of data and greater variety of persepectives than the same time spent in an in-depth interview. However, the group environment has a more valuable contribution than simply generating a large volume of data; it is the interaction between group members that leads to the unique type of data found in focus group research. The group environment enables participants to raise different perspectives and discuss issues with relatively little moderator involvement, thereby identifying new issues or perspectives on the research topic that may be unanticipated by the researcher. Furthermore, the discussion element allows participants to build on the responses of others, provide contrasting views, and debate issues, thereby producing a different type of data that reveals participants' insights about an issue that is beyond what may be contributed by a single interviewee alone. Group interaction also influences the quality of data produced. Participants are able to react to the contributions of others in the group, which may lead to reflection, justification, or refinement of comments made during the discussion, providing a clearer and potentially deeper understanding of the issues discussed. In addition, the group environment acts to temper extreme views within the group, and is therefore a highly effective method to access community norms, views, and behavior. This social moderation of information results from the group nature of data collection and is therefore not evident in individual interviews.

A further advantage of the group setting is that it creates a comfortable environment for participants to discuss issues and may encourage reluctant participants to share their views. The group setting may make participants feel less threatened to share negative views, compared with an individual interview setting, because the negative views or criticisms are seen as a product of the group rather than an individual per se (Green & Thorogood, 2004). For example, when participants hear that others in the group have criticisms of a community service they may be more inclined to share their own criticisms of the service. Furthermore, a reluctant participant may be more inclined to share their views when they can hear the experiences of others that may align with their own experience or stimulate them to share their unique perspectives. For these participants the group setting can "break the ice," whereas they may remain more reluctant in a one-on-one interview setting (Liamputtong & Ezzy, 2007).

Many of the limitations of focus group research are the inverse of the advantages of the method, and are summarized in Figure 1.4. Many of these limitations can be managed with careful attention to planning and conducting the group discussions, as described in Chapter 2.

One challenge in conducting focus group discussions is that the fluid nature of a group discussion can lead to a less controlled environment for data collection. This requires a skilled and experienced moderator to facilitate the discussion and manage the group dynamics to generate useful data. Using an unskilled moderator can easily lead to the collection of redundant or superficial information. A moderator also needs to ask open, neutral questions yet keep the discussion focused on the research topics. Morgan (1997, p. 14) states that "there is a very real concern that the moderator, in the name of maintaining the interview's focus, will influence the group's interactions." Therefore, an inexperienced moderator may inadvertently bias the contributions of participants, reducing the quality and validity of data collected. Identifying a skilled moderator is a core challenge in using this method, particularly when group discussions are held in another language where moderators often need to be quickly identified, briefed, and trained for the task.

A second limitation of focus group research is managing the group dynamics. With a group of participants there is always a risk that someone will dominate the discussion thereby stifling the contributions of others. Another issue that may develop is "group talk," whereby participants may conform to what others have said even though they may not actually agree. This may be a result of social pressure to conform or because of the development of a hierarchy in the group. These situations lead to the absence of discussion, a lack of diversity in the discussion, and ultimately a reduction in data quality. An experienced moderator is therefore critical to manage these group dynamics to make participants feel comfortable enough to contribute to the discussion. Some issues with group dynamics are caused by poor recruitment of participants. In particular a lack of heterogeneity among group members can lead to the formation of a hierarchy, which can also impact participants' willingness to contribute to the discussion. A further limitation of the group setting is the reduced confidentiality compared with an individual interview. This may lead some participants to withhold certain information in the group and reduce the depth of information received on some issues (David & Sutton, 2004).

There are also limitations in the data that are collected in a group setting. A focus group discussion can only cover a limited number of topics, because there needs to be sufficient time for participants to contribute and for a discussion on each issue. Therefore, focus group discussions may not provide in-depth data to the same extent as an individual interview (Krueger & Casey, 2009; Hopkins, 2007). It must also be remembered that focus group data are a product of an interactive discussion and responses are not independent of the influence of other participants. Therefore, focus group discussions are not suitable for collecting data on individual perspectives. Furthermore, although focus group discussions are well suited for identifying normative behavior, they are less useful for identifying marginal behavior because participants may not be willing to share experiences that differ from the social norm in a group setting (Green & Thorogood, 2004).

Finally, focus group discussions generate a large volume of data and data analysis can be time consuming. In addition, data analysis can be complex because it needs to account for the context of the group discussion whereby participants may change their views or provide contradictory opinions during the course of the discussion (Hennink, 2007). Finally, focus group research is not cheap and quick (Morgan, 1997; Morgan & Krueger, 1993) as is popularly believed. It requires a great deal of time to collect, manage, and analyze the data, which therefore becomes costly.

Key Points

....

- A focus group discussion is a qualitative research method involving an interactive discussion and led by a trained moderator.
- The essential purpose of a focus group discussion is to identify a range of views on the research topic, and to gain an understanding of these issues from the perspective of participants themselves.
- Focus group discussions use non-directive interviewing, which involves generating data from a discussion between participants and gives participants greater control of the issues raised.
- An interactive discussion between participants leads to the unique data produced, which is not found by interviewing an individual participant.
- The group environment acts to temper extreme views and is highly effective for identifying community norms.
- There exist different applications of focus group discussions, each with variation in their purpose, procedure, and outcome.

- Focus group discussions can be used for behavioral research, evaluating social programs, developing public policy, designing health promotion strategies, and conducting needs assessments.
- Focus group discussions may be used for exploratory, explanatory, or evaluation research; and are effective in mixed methods research designs.
- The group environment of data collection has advantages and limitations. Therefore, a skilled moderator is needed to conduct the group discussion and manage group dynamics.

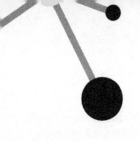

DESIGNING AND CONDUCTING FOCUS GROUP RESEARCH

2

THERE IS NO definitive correct way to conduct focus group research. Each study is shaped by the specific research question, theoretical framework, study context, and characteristics of the study participants. In addition, practical realities, such as the time-frame and funding of a study, and unique field challenges influence the methodological decisions of a study. Therefore, focus group research can vary. Despite some variability in application, there are some general guidelines and important considerations in conducting focus group research that can improve methodological rigor and therefore the quality of data produced.

This chapter provides guidance on planning and conducting focus group discussions. It describes tasks in preparing for focus group research, such as training the field team, recruiting participants, developing questions for the discussion guide, and ethical considerations. The chapter then focuses on conducting focus group discussions, describing the role of the moderator in conducting the discussion, managing group dynamics, and promoting an interactive discussion. Finally, a brief overview of approaches to analyzing focus group data is given. Each of these tasks is described concisely; however, further readings are provided for additional guidance.

Planning Focus Group Research

Training the Field Team

A focus group team typically consists of a moderator and note-taker. However, some studies may have a larger field team including several moderators, particularly when both male and female moderators are needed, or transcribers. Often members of a field team conduct multiple tasks, where possible.

Regardless of the size of a focus group team, training is essential. However, this task is often overlooked when planning focus group research. Training all team members on the goals of the study, fieldwork protocols, and specific tasks they will conduct is important to ensure consistency in all field tasks. Not all team members will be familiar with the methodological approach of focus group discussions or they may have used a different application of the method (e.g., market research or participatory approaches, see chapter 1), it is therefore necessary to brief team members on how focus group discussions are conducted in academic research. Training becomes particularly important in international research where moderators may have been recruited for their language skills and thus not be familiar with how to conduct qualitative research or focus group discussions in particular.

The content of the training sessions is guided by the research skills and experience of team members recruited. Training often includes a briefing on the study objectives, focus group research, and ethical issues, and then more detailed training on the research instrument itself, strategies for group moderation, transcription, and (if needed) translation protocols. It is useful to train team members on all the different fieldwork roles, not only the specific tasks they will conduct. This enables team members to interchange roles if needed and maintains consistency between these roles. For moderating a group discussion, training needs to include strategies for developing rapport, impartial moderation, managing group dynamics, fostering discussion, effective listening, probing, and pacing a discussion. For the role of note-taking during the group discussion, training needs to include objective note-taking and strategies for paraphrasing main points, noting key phrases, recording body language, and structuring written notes. In addition, a note-taker is usually responsible for operating the recording device. For transcribing the recording of the group discussions, training is needed on developing a verbatim record of the discussion; structuring transcripts; and translation protocols (if needed).

It can be extremely valuable to include role-play activities as part of the training sessions. This may involve practicing group moderation skills (particularly probing); note-taking; and verbatim transcription. Observing role-play is a useful strategy for providing tangible feedback on improving skills. Figure 2.1 shows a field team in Burkina Faso listening to the recording of a focus group discussion and practicing verbatim transcription. For further instruction on training field teams see Hennink (2007).

Focus Group Size and Composition

A focus group discussion typically includes six to eight participants. It needs to be "small enough for everyone to have an opportunity to share insights and yet large enough to provide diversity of perceptions" (Krueger & Casey, 2000, p. 10). With fewer than six participants less diversity is captured in the group discussion and with greater than eight participants it becomes difficult for a moderator to manage a productive discussion.

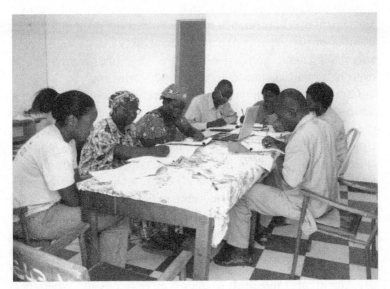

Photo: M. Hennink

Figure 2.1. Field team training on verbatim transcription in Burkina Faso.

The size of a focus group is also influenced by the purpose of the study, the topic of discussion, and the type of participants. A group of six participants may be suitable if the research topic is intense or participants have much experience on the topic, whereby each participant is likely to have a lot to contribute to the discussion. The drawback of a smaller group is the limited diversity of experience shared; even six participants have a limited pool of experience and contributions. A small group of participants also loses some of the interactive dynamics of a group discussion (Smithson, 2008) because there are fewer people to respond to issues raised. In addition, smaller groups are more easily affected by group dynamics. For example, if there are one or two dominant participants it has a greater impact in a smaller group and the issues discussed are more likely to reflect the views of those dominant members (Ulin, Robinson, Tolley, & McNeill, 2002; Bloor, Frankland, Thomas, Robson, 2001). Small groups can be well justified when study participants are children. Gibson (2007) recommends a group size of four to five participants who have only a 1–2 year age range when conducting focus groups with children. Larger focus groups of eight participants are more common and are suitable where the topic of discussion is broad, or where participants may have less specific experience on the research topic. In these situations each participant may contribute less to the discussion, justifying a larger number of participants to capture diversity in views and experiences. Whichever group size is desired, it is usually advisable to overrecruit participants to account for any attrition.

Group composition refers to the characteristics of participants in a focus group. Group composition can have a significant effect on the group dynamics during a discussion and therefore needs careful consideration. Effective group composition can create a comfortable, permissive environment that fosters productive discussion. Poor group composition can quickly create an uncomfortable environment where participants become reluctant to contribute to the discussion thereby reducing the quality of data generated.

Two aspects of group composition are important for developing a positive group environment: homogeneity between participants and their level of acquaintance. Homogeneity is desired because participants are more likely to share their opinions and experiences with others who they perceive are similar to them, whereas they will be reluctant to contribute if they believe others in the group differ from them in terms of status or knowledge. Homogeneity among participants therefore fosters an open productive discussion, which contributes to better quality data. Conradson (2005, p. 133) states that group homogeneity involves "bringing together people who have enough in common to allow the development of a productive conversational dynamic."

Group homogeneity is generally sought in the socio-cultural backgrounds of participants or their level of experience with the study topic (not in their opinions of the discussion issues). Perhaps the most common strategy to achieve homogeneity is to segment focus groups by gender and age group (e.g., by conducting separate group discussion with participants who are young women, older women, young men, and older men). This stratification makes sense for many studies and often no further homogeneity is needed. Stratifying groups by these characteristics is also advantageous for data analysis, whereby issues raised can be compared by age and gender of participants to identify any patterns. It is common practice to conduct separate focus groups by gender, because it remains unclear how a mixed-gender group composition affects participant's contributions to the discussion (Fern, 2001; Morgan, 1997). It is also advisable to avoid a group composition with participants from vastly different socioeconomic groups, life stages, or levels of authority because this can quickly create a hierarchy in the group, which can inhibit some members from contributing to the discussion. Although group homogeneity in demographic characteristics is desirable, too much specificity (beyond age and gender) makes participant recruitment challenging and leads to too many groups. Group homogeneity can also be achieved among participants who share the same intense experience (e.g., women who experienced multiple births or people with a severe illness). Sharing similar experiences often creates a strong shared identity among participants that overrides the need to create homogeneity through demographic characteristics.

The level of acquaintance between participants can also influence group participation. Focus groups may be held among a group of strangers or with participants who are familiar to one another. Both types of group composition can be effective. However, one needs to be aware of the potential effects that the level of acquaintance can have on a group discussion. Recruiting a group of strangers for a focus group discussion is often a preferred strategy because there are fewer issues to manage. Among strangers there is greater anonymity, which may increase a participant's willingness to contribute to the discussion. A group of strangers may also provide more detailed contributions to the discussion because they need to provide more context or explanation of their views, whereas a group of people who are familiar with one another may already know a participant's viewpoint and reasoning on certain issues, and therefore less detail is given. The main drawbacks of recruiting a group of strangers are the potential for non-attendance and the longer time needed to develop group rapport compared with participants who are already acquainted. It is also advisable that the moderator and note-taker are not familiar to participants because they may be associated with particular points of view that influence participant's contribution to the discussion. In some study contexts, recruiting a group of strangers is difficult, for example conducting focus group discussion in urban slums or high-density neighborhoods where most people know one another. In these situations familiarity can be reduced by ensuring that close neighbors or family members are not present in the same focus group discussion (see Hennink 2007 for further guidance on recruiting participants in international focus group research).

Focus groups may also comprise participants who are well acquainted, such as members of the same social network, therapy group, or exercise class. For example, Koppelman and Bourjolly (2001) conducted focus group discussions among women with severe psychiatric disabilities who were part of the same mental health women's group, to facilitate their comfort in discussing living with their conditions. The advantage of recruiting a group of acquaintances is that less time needed to build group rapport because participants are already familiar to one another. Group attendance may also be greater because participants may know others attending the group discussion so there may be less attrition. One of the main issues with pre-existing groups is the level of shared knowledge participants have about each other. This can be an advantage in that other group members will add detail to a point made by another speaker, thereby increasing the depth and potential accuracy of information gathered. However, there is also the risk of overdisclosure and reduced confidentiality if the speaker preferred that the additional details were not shared with the group. Familiarity among group members can also lead to participants providing overall less detail in their contributions simply because others in the group already know their perspectives or because of a concern that group members may share their views with others in their shared social network. Therefore, the lack of anonymity among acquaintance groups may reduce the depth of information provided compared with a group of strangers.

Recruiting Participants

In qualitative research the purpose of participant recruitment is different from quantitative studies. Quantitative research typically seeks to measure issues and extrapolate the study findings to the general population; therefore, a large sample size and random selection of participants is required. However, the aim of qualitative research is entirely different. The purpose of focus group research is "not to infer but to understand, not to generalize but determine the range, and not to make statements about the population but to provide insights about how people in the groups perceive a situation" (Krueger & Casey, 2009, p. 66). This not only requires a small number of study participants so that issues can be explored in depth, but also necessitates identifying participants with specific characteristics to best inform the research issues rather than selecting them randomly. Furthermore, focus group research seeks not only normative views but often actively seeks the perspectives of "outliers" or deviant behavior to enable the full range of behaviors or perceptions on the research issues to be captured. This requires a different approach to participant recruitment than that used in quantitative studies. Therefore, recruiting a large sample or seeking random selection of participants is not appropriate for focus group research, and does not improve the quality of a study.

Qualitative research uses purposive (or nonrandom) methods of participant recruitment. Participants in qualitative research are selected "on purpose" because they have specific characteristics or experience that can best inform the research issues. These are often referred to as "information rich" participants. For example, a study on the experiences of young parenthood may seek to recruit adolescent parents because they are "information rich" on the experience of being very young parents. Selecting participants with specific characteristics requires a non-random method of participant recruitment because people with the required characteristics are unlikely to be evenly distributed in the population and likely to be missed if random selection was used. Purposive recruitment also begins to theorize about which dimensions (e.g., demographic, experiential, or geographic) may influence different perspectives on the research issues, so that these can be built into the participant recruitment structure. For example, conducting separate group discussions in rural and urban areas begins to anticipate potentially fruitful differences that may arise on the research issues during data analysis. Purposive recruitment adds strength to focus group research; it enables recruitment to be focused and deliberate, and should not be seen as haphazard or conducted without principles or procedure (Hennink, Hutter, & Bailey, 2011).

Purposive recruitment is iterative, whereby it can evolve during the research process. Initially the study population is defined at the outset of the study and then refined it in an iterative way during data collection. The study population is first defined during the research design process, where the research question, academic literature, and theory help refine the most appropriate study population. At this stage segmentation of the study population may be identified, whereby separate focus groups are conducted with different types of study participants, such as service users and non-users, or different types of participants (e.g., patients, doctors, and health insurers). It is important that the study population be clearly defined at the outset, to determine who is eligible to participate in the study and to identify the most suitable method of participant recruitment. As data collection begins and one learns more about the research issues, other types of study participants may be identified to include in the study. This may involve broadening or narrowing the original study population or adding specific subgroups of participants who may provide useful perspectives on the research issues but were not considered at the outset of the research. For example, a study on encouraging cycling to work may initially recruit only those who cycle to identify their perspectives, but during data collection it is revealed that workplace policies and infrastructure (e.g., cycle racks, lockers, showers, and so forth) are strong motivators for cycling to work and therefore decide to recruit workplace managers to the participant pool to explore the workplace policy issues on cycling. In this way, the participant pool expands in an inductive way informed by data collection, to add specific types of participants who may add valuable perspectives on the research issues.

Qualitative research typically includes a small number of study participants to achieve depth of information and variation of perspectives. The number of participants to include in a study is guided by the principle of saturation (Glaser & Strauss, 1967). This is the point at which information collected begins to repeat itself. After reaching the point of saturation, any additional data collection becomes redundant, because the purpose of qualitative research is to uncover diversity and context, rather than a large number of participants with the same type of experience. For example, if conducting a study on men's motivations for getting health screening and after the second focus group discussion 10 different motivations for health screening have been identified in detail, and in the third focus group discussion the same motivations are repeated, then the point of information saturation has been reached, whereby no more new information is being identified. Further data collection is now redundant because the diversity of motivations among men has been identified and additional data collection would provide no further understanding of the issue. Repetition of issues is therefore an indicator of saturation. It is also important to check that there is diversity in the study population so that issues are captured among rural men, urban men, older and younger men, and so on. If the study population is segmented (e.g., by older/younger or urban/rural participants), it is good practice to conduct at least two groups, but preferably more, with each sub-group of participants to assess saturation within each sub-group. Including diversity in the study population and allowing saturation to be reached through the iterative process increases the validity of data collected.

The number of focus groups to conduct is therefore determined through an iterative process until information saturation is reached. This process can only begin after data collection is initiated, which can be problematic because researchers often need to indicate the number of focus group discussions to conduct in the research proposal (before any data collection). It is therefore necessary to predetermine the number of focus group discussions needed to reach saturation on the study topic. This can be done by considering the nature of the study topic (broad or narrow); the type of research (exploratory or specific); the diversity or segmentation of the study population; and the resources available for the study. If the study is exploratory and the topic is broad more groups may be needed to capture diversity of issues and reach saturation. If the study population is segmented, more groups are needed to reach saturation. Given the range of influences in estimating saturation, the number of focus groups can vary widely between studies. Ritchie and Lewis (2003) suggest that many studies have less than 20 focus group discussions. However, what is more important than the actual number of study participants, is how the number of participants is determined and justified for each study (Hennink et al., 2011).

There are many strategies for purposive recruitment of participants in qualitative research. Some effective strategies for recruiting focus group participants are summarized in the table below. For further details on each strategy see Hennink et al. (2011). No single recruitment strategy is completely ideal; each strategy has strengths and limitations. Often several recruitment strategies are used in a single study or different recruitment strategies are used for different types of study participants. For example, different recruitment strategies may be used in rural and urban study sites or for younger and older participants.

Participant Recruitment Strategies

Community Gatekeepers	Community gatekeepers facilitate access to the study population. They may be social or religious leaders, service providers, or familiar and respected members of the study community. Community gatekeeper may be asked to contact eligible study participants and refer them to the study or to attend an informational presentation about the study. Gatekeepers provide trusted access to the study population, therefore their involvement in participant recruitment can significantly increase participation.

Formal Services	Identify whether the study population regularly uses any formal services or networks (e.g., health services, religious groups, or support groups) from which they may be recruited. These services can then be used to provide information about the study in flyers posted at the venues, by giving a presentation about the study, or by asking service staff to refer eligible people to the study. Alternatively, people can be intercepted as they exit a service to invite their participation in a focus group discussion.
Informal Networks	Identify whether the study population is associated with any informal networks, such as social or recreation groups (e.g., sports clubs, youth groups, language classes). These networks can be used to inform potential participants about the study and invite their participation in a focus group.
Advertisements	Develop an advertisement about the study to place in newspapers, magazines, community bulletin boards, or other prominent locations likely to be viewed by the study population. This strategy is most useful for "hard to reach" study populations and requires significant incentives for people to attend the group discussion.
Research-based	In mixed-methods research, focus group participants may be recruited from the pool of study participants recruited for another part of the study. For example, if a study includes a quantitative survey then focus group participants may be recruited from survey respondents. One advantage of this method is that information from the survey can be used to refine the purposive selection of participants with specific characteristics.

Ethical Issues

Ethics are a set of moral principles that researchers abide by to protect study participants from harm by researchers or the research process. Codes of research ethics are comprised of informed consent, self-determination, minimization of harm, anonymity, and confidentiality (see the *Declaration of Helsinki* (World Medical association 2008) and *Belmont Report* (National Comission for the Protection of Human Subjects of Behavioral Research (1978) for fuller descriptions of each). It is critical to consider ethical issues that may arise in focus group research when planning to use this method. Even though ethical approval may have been granted at the beginning of a study, attention to ethical issues does not stop there. The study still needs to be conducted in an ethical way and ethical challenges need to be managed. Focus group research requires continual assessment of ethical issues because of the evolving nature of data collection. This means that researchers need to remain continually mindful of ethical issues that may arise as the study evolves. In addition, focus group research poses ethical challenges because of the intense interaction with study participants and the group nature of data collection, as described next.

"Self-determination" refers to participants' right to determine whether they wish to participate in the study and their right to refuse participation without any negative consequences. This requires "informed consent," whereby focus group participants are provided with sufficient, relevant, and accurate information about the study, in a comprehensible format, so that they can make an informed decision on whether or not to participate in a group discussion. Participants should be provided with information about the study, what their participation will involve, any potential risks or benefits from participation, and how data will be used and safeguarded. They should also be informed that if they participate in the study they do not have to answer any questions if they prefer not to, and that they are free to leave the discussion at any time. Seeking informed consent is often done initially during participant recruitment and reinforced again during the moderator's introduction at the beginning of the group discussion. Central to informed consent is that participation is voluntary and not coerced. In some communities, participation in the group discussion may be authorized by others, such as household elders or a community leader. It should not be assumed that a participant has consented to participate in the group discussion and individual consent should always be sought. Seeking written consent is common; however, oral consent may be more appropriate in some circumstances, such as among a study population with low literacy. Researchers also need to seek consent for recording the group discussion and in doing so describe why a recording is needed, and how it will be used and safeguarded.

There is a responsibility to minimize any potential risks to participants from their involvement in the study. Harm can take many forms: physical harm, such as violence from others finding out what was disclosed in the discussion; social harm, whereby a participant's reputation in the community is damaged from their association with the study; psychological harm, such as embarrassment or judgment from others in the group; or economic harm, through loss of wages while attending the group discussion. Researchers have an obligation to reduce any such harm to participants and inform them of any potential risks from participating in the study. Care also needs to be taken in the provision of incentives to participants, to ensure that the incentive is not coercive whereby a participant may undertake some risks to be involved in the study to receive the incentive.

Finally, it is the researcher's responsibility to keep confidential the information discussed in the focus group and to maintain anonymity of group participants. It is difficult to ensure complete confidentiality in a focus group discussion because the information is discussed in a group setting and one cannot ensure that participants will not disclose the content of the discussion with others outside the group. This is particularly problematic when focus groups are conducted among acquaintances who share the same social or professional network. There is also the risk of overdisclosure whereby participants who are familiar to one another may reveal information about others in the group that they themselves would not have disclosed. This puts the onus on a moderator to reinforce issues of confidentiality to the group and encourage participants not to divulge what was discussed outside the group. Researchers can, however, restrict who listens to the recording of the discussion and store data securely to maintain confidentiality of the information discussed. The dynamic nature of a focus group discussion also means that the discussion may flow into other topics that were not outlined by the moderator in the introduction and participants need to be made aware of the fluid nature of the discussion. In addition, confidentiality can be difficult to maintain because researchers use quotations from study participants when reporting the study findings. This tradition underscores the need to ensure anonymity of data by removing any identifiable information from the transcript of the group discussion and ensure that quotations are reported in a way that does not disclose the identity of individual participants. The names of participants, if these were collected, should always be kept secure to protect the identities of participants and participants need to be informed how their identity will be protected.

Developing the Discussion Guide

A discussion guide is a pre-prepared list of topics or actual questions used by a moderator to guide the group discussion. A discussion guide can seem deceptively simple; however, it requires considerable forethought to develop an effective guide that fosters productive discussion and elicits useful information to meet the research objectives. Designing a discussion guide is one of the key tasks in preparing for focus group research.

A discussion guide has several functions. Its main purpose is to remind the moderator of the topics and questions that need to be covered to meet the research objectives. Although the questions on the discussion guide are structured in a logical sequence, the actual discussion may proceed in a more haphazard manner as the moderator follows issues raised spontaneously by participants. Therefore, "the moderator uses the guide as a resource to maintain the balance between the researchers focus and the group's discussion" (Morgan, 1997, p. 48). The discussion guide thus becomes a checklist to ensure that all topics were covered by the close of the discussion. The discussion guide also assists the moderator to manage the group discussion by providing effective "warm-up" questions to build rapport and "closing" questions to signal the discussion is coming to an end. It can also include prompts, instructions, and reminders for the moderator (e.g., a reminder to cover ethical issues, indicate where to do a group activity, or to thank participants and provide gifts at the end). A further function of the discussion guide is to introduce some consistency in the data collected among different focus groups in the study, which is particularly beneficial if several moderators are used. This enables a comparison of issues across groups to be made during data analysis. This is not to suggest that each moderator needs to ask questions in the same order, but that the same topics or questioning strategies are used across each group so that the results are comparable.

A discussion guide may take different formats, ranging from a simple list of topics to more fully developed questions and probes. A topic guide consists of a list of topics to be covered during the group discussion from which the moderator formulates impromptu questions during the discussion itself. It is generally quick to develop and may lead to a more informal style of questioning. However, there is a great deal of pressure on the moderator to formulate questions on each topic as the discussion progresses, which requires an experienced moderator. A further limitation is the potential lack of consistency in questions asked between different groups particularly where several moderators are used, thereby reducing comparability in data analysis (Hennink, 2007). Furthermore, a topic guide also cannot be pilot tested to check the effectiveness of a questioning strategy, because the actual questions are developed spontaneously by the moderator during the discussion. In academic research the discussion guide is often more fully developed including pre-designed questions and probes. Although this type of discussion guide takes time to develop it overcomes the need for a moderator to formulate impromptu questions, and provides greater consistency in the questions asked across groups. These are important benefits for academic research, where the study population is often divided into subgroups and the issues compared between groups. One drawback may be the reduced spontaneity in the delivery of questions, although an experienced moderator can easily develop a more informal style of questioning using a pre-prepared discussion guide. Krueger (1998) provides a more detailed discussion of these different types of discussion guides. Some moderators may use no discussion guide at all, because they believe it imposes too much structure to the flow of a natural discussion (Greenbaum, 2000). However, "experienced moderators understand the benefits of using a discussion guide in providing structure and focus to the group discussion, while at the same time not feeling constrained by the guide when following new or interesting issues in the discussion" (Hennink, 2007, p. 49). Whichever type of discussion guide is used, it should be seen as a guide, not a rigid format, that helps the moderator focus the discussion while also maintaining the flexibility to change the topic order or explore new issues as they arise in the discussion.

A discussion guide is not a static research instrument. It often is moderately refined during the process of data collection as more is learned about the study topic. These modifications typically involve refining existing questions, adding more specific probes, or adding additional questions on new issues identified during data collection. The broad structure and focus of the discussion guide usually remains the same throughout the research process, but the refinements add focus, which allows an exploration of issues in greater depth in each subsequent group discussion. For example, a discussion guide may ask a question on the cost of a specific health treatment, whereby participants indicate that they can afford the treatment cost but the frequent clinic visits lead to high transport costs that are not manegable. In light of this information the discussion guide may be modified to add a specific probe about transport costs, thereby enabling researchers to use inductive leads from one group discussion to go deeper into the issues in subsequent groups and more fully explore the issues. Some consistency in the discussion guide is important because one needs to identify when saturation has been reached and data collection should cease, which is only possible with broad consistency in questioning.

Structure of the Discussion Guide

The structure of the discussion guide is important. It can assist the moderator to manage the group discussion by effectively opening the discussion, focusing on key topics, and bringing the discussion to a close (Hennink et al., 2011).

A discussion guide should have a clear and logical structure, even though the actual discussion may follow a different order. The sequence of questions and topics should make sense for the participants, so that a smooth discussion may follow with limited redundancy or repetition of issues. For example, if the discussion focuses on the process of migration, it makes sense to begin by asking about issues before migration, then ask about the actual migration, followed by questions about the postmigration experience. However, remember that once the group discussion is underway the order in which topics arise may differ from how they appear on the discussion guide. Nonetheless, a logically ordered guide can help the moderator to memorize the questioning structure, which can be useful during an active discussion to recall topics covered and those to still pursue.

An effective structure follows an hourglass design as depicted in Figure 2.2. The basic principle is to begin the discussion with broad questions to build rapport among group participants so that they begin to feel comfortable in the group environment before moving on to discuss the more specific topics that are critical to meet the research objectives, and then move again to broader summary issues to end the discussion. Each part of the hourglass structure has a specific purpose. The wide top of the hourglass depicts the broad introduction given to participants to provide cognition so they know what to expect during the group discussion. The opening questions begin to develop rapport with participants and make them feel comfortable in the group environment. As the hourglass narrows the discussion guide moves

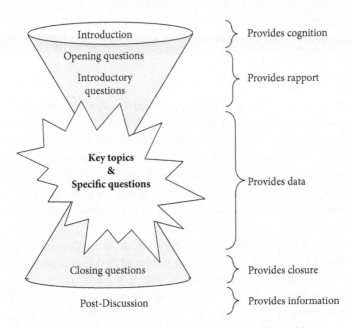

Figure 2.2. Hourglass design of the focus group discussion guide.

toward more specific questions that provide data to respond to the research questions. A discussion guide may include several topics with a series of specific questions under each topic. These topics are placed in the center of the discussion guide so that there is sufficient time for participants to feel comfortable in contributing to the discussion before asking these questions, thereby improving data quality. These specific questions typically comprise one-half to two-thirds of the discussion guide. The hourglass then begins to widen again, depicting a move back toward broad questions that provide closure to the discussion. Closing questions indicate that the discussion is coming to an end and can be immensely helpful for wrapping up an active discussion. In some cases there may also be a post-discussion stage whereby participants are provided with information or resources or asked to complete a deomgraphic survey.

A typical discussion guide includes the following components: an introduction, an opening question, a series of short introductory questions, transitions questions or statements, key topics with specific questions, and closing questions. These components (based on Krueger & Casey, 2009) each have a different purpose as described next. An example discussion guide that includes these components is shown in Figure 2.3 from a study among adolescents attending a summer camp for overweight children.

Introduction

A focus group discussion typically begins with an introduction by the moderator, which may be included in the discussion guide as a written narrative or a series of bullet points. The moderator's introduction begins the process of rapport development and should therefore be given in a friendly informal way to make participants feel at ease, rather than reading a formal statement. An introduction script is shown in the example discussion guide in Figure 2.3.

During the introduction the moderator conducts a number of tasks. The moderator should first welcome and thank participants for attending the discussion, and may ask participants to introduce themselves. A note-taker should also be introduced, so that participants are aware of their role. It can be helpful to indicate why participants were selected for the study (e.g., they may share

Introduction

Thank you all for coming today. My name is (moderator) and this is (note-taker). We are helping (health agency) to find out about your experiences of this summer camp and how it can be improved. The best way to do this is to talk to people who attended the camp, so we are holding these discussion groups with boys and girls at the camp this week. In our discussion today we just want to talk about your experiences at this camp, what you did here, what you learned, what you liked and didn't like – all to help improve the experience for the next camp.

We are not part of the camp itself and are just collecting the information, so we hope that you will feel comfortable to share with us what you really thought about this camp. Please don't feel shy, we want to hear from all of you about your time here. You are the experts because you have been at camp this week and we are here to learn from you. There are no right or wrong answers we simply want to hear your thoughts and suggestions. I have some questions for you but also feel free to add other things you feel are important as we go along.

During our discussion (note-taker) will be taking notes and reminding me if I forget to ask something, but s/he cannot write down every word we say so we would like to record the discussion so that we don't miss anything that is said. Please don't be concerned about this, our discussion will stay confidential and only the research team will listen to the recording. Camp leaders will not listen to the recording. **Is it OK with everyone to record the discussion?**

During our discussion please let everyone share their views, but only one person should speak at a time so that the recording will be clear. Just join in when you have something to say, we will not be going around the group for every question. Remember we want to hear all your views. It's OK to disagree with others if you have a different opinion but please also respect other people's views. Also, everything that you hear today should be confidential and not shared with people who are outside the group. This discussion will last about one hour, please help yourself to the refreshments. **Are there any questions before we start?**

Figure 2.3. Example focus group discussion guide.

Let's start by introducing ourselves....

1. Let's each share our first names and where you are from.

2. What type of summer camps have you all been to before? (probe: activities, location)

EXPECTATIONS ABOUT CAMP

First, I would like to hear about your expectations before you came to this camp...

3. What made you all chose to come to this camp? (probe: parents, friends, activities, cost)

4. What did you expect this camp would be like before you came? (probe: people, activities, lessons)
   a) What were you most excited about?
   b) What were you most worried about?

5. How was the camp different to what you expected?

HEALTHY LIFESTYLE LESSONS LEARNED

Now let's focus on what you did and learned at this summer camp...

6. What new things did you learn here about having a healthy lifestyle? (probe on four lifestyle lessons)

7. Which healthy habits from camp can you manage back at home? (probe: reasons)

8. Which healthy habits would be hard to keep at home? (probe: reasons)

ASSESSMENT OF CAMP

Now let's talk about all the things you liked and didn't like about this summer camp...

9. What did you like most about this camp? (probe: activities, people, camp leaders)

10. What were the things you didn't like about this camp? (probe: reasons why)

Figure 2.3. (Continued)

a) How could these things be changed for future camps?

11. What was the <u>hardest thing</u> you did this week? (probe: physical activity, restrict diet, no cellphones)

SUMMARY & CLOSING

I just have a few last questions....

12. How could more people be encouraged to come to this camp?

13. What would you tell your friends who are considering coming to this camp?

14. Of all the things we discussed today, which are the <u>three most</u> important things to improve this summer camp?

Are there any other things about this camp that you would like to share before we finish?

Thank you for sharing your thoughts with us today

Figure 2.3. (Continued)

a common experience or be residents of the same neighborhood). This reinforces homogeneity among participants, which makes people feel at ease and encourages participation in the discussion. A brief summary of the study is generally provided, as is an indication about how the information will be used. Ethical issues also need to be reviewed during the introduction. Although permissions may have been sought before participants joined the group, a moderator often reviews permission to record the discussion, emphasising that participation is voluntary, and ensuring participants of confidentiality of the discussion.

Finally, the moderator needs to outline how the group discussion will be conducted. This provides participants with cognition, so they know what to expect and feel confident to contribute to the discussion (Hennink & Diamond, 1999). Participants should be encouraged to speak at any time, but that only one person should speak at a time so all dialogue is clearly captured on the recording. It should be stressed that there are no right or wrong answers, that individual views are important and different views are valuable, and that it is acceptable to disagree with others in the group who may have different opinions. The moderator can also indicate that they are not an expert in the topic and their role is to facilitate the discussion among the participants who are most knowledgeable about the issues. Participants should also be encouraged to share their comments with the whole group rather than the person seated next to them to discourage fragmentation of the discussion. The length of the session needs to be indicated at the beginning of the discussion. Many moderators also request that cell phones be turned to silent mode.

Opening Question

The first question on the discussion guide is the opening question. It is usually a simple question that all participants can respond to and begins to make participants feel comfortable to contribute to the discussion. The opening question is not intended to promote discussion, therefore it is often short and factual. For example, "Let's start with everyone telling the group which study program you are enrolled in and when you expect to graduate." Some moderators prefer to go around the group allowing each person to respond to the opening question. A subtle benefit of this strategy is that it allows each person to say something at the begining of the discussion, which can promote contribution throughout the discussion, because the longer one remains silent in a group the more reluctant they may be to contribute later in the discussion (Hennink, 2007; Ritchie & Lewis, 2003). The opening question is not intended to produce data and the information is rarely analyzed.

Another strategy for opening the discussion is to conduct a brief activity. For example, Kitzinger (1994) used pile-sorting as an opening activity in a focus group discussion about media images related to AIDS. Participants were asked to sort images into piles according to criteria given by the moderator, for example whether the group believed the images were effective or offensive. Similarly, Hesse-Biber and Leavy (2006) conducted group discussions among gay men, whereby the opening strategy involved the moderator reading a paragraph-long quotation to the group and asking for their reactions. This began an in-depth dialogue that led to many of the issues on the discussion guide. Using an activity can take time and reduces the actual discussion time; therefore, it needs to be clearly related to the study topic whereby it can simultaneously build rapport and generate data, as in the examples described.

Introductory Questions

Introductory questions act as a "warm up" for the discussion and begin to focus participants' attention on the research issues. They typically comprise a series of questions with the moderator asking impromptu follow-up questions to encourage detailed responses from participants. It is useful to include several introductory questions, because it can take 10–15 minutes for participants to feel comfortable in a group discussion. An example of a series of introductory questions for a discussion on physical activity among the elderly may be as follows:

1. What types of physical activities are common among the elderly in this community?
2. Where do elderly people generally go to exercise?
3. With whom do elderly people usually exercise?
4. What type of elderly people exercise regularly?

An alternative introductory strategy is to ask the group to explain a term or phrase that is central to the research topic. For example, "We often hear the term 'glass ceiling' in relation to the promotion of women in the workforce, what does this term mean to you?" or "What does a 'balanced diet' mean?" These types of introductory questions provide the group with a common knowledge base about the term or phrase from which the moderator can then build the discussion.

Transition Statements

Transition statements signal a change between topics in the discussion guide. They may be used multiple times throughout the discussion, in particular when transitioning between the key topics and into the closing questions. Several transition statements are shown in the discussion guide in Figure 2.3. For example, the statement "First, I would like to hear about your expectations before you came to this camp" provides a transition between the introductory questions and the first key topic about participant's expectations of the camp. Similarly, the statement "Now let's talk about all the things you liked and didn't like about this summer camp" signals a move to a new topic about assessing the camp experience.

Key Questions

Key questions are the most important part of the discussion guide. They are the essential questions that generate data to meet the research objectives. This section may include a series of individual questions or several topics each containing a series of questions as shown in the example in Figure 2.3. Key questions include more probes than other parts of the discussion guide to generate detailed responses and promote a discussion on these critical issues. Key questions are placed about one-third to halfway through the discussion guide when participants are warmed up and comfortable in the group setting. At least half of the discussion time is allocated to the key questions. These questions generate the core study data and are therefore analyzed in the greatest depth. The section below on "question design" provides guidance on developing effective questions for this section of the discussion guide.

Closing Questions

Closing questions are designed to signal that the discussion is coming to an end. They help the moderator to effectively close the discussion, but can also provide valuable information that summarizes the issues discussed and can therefore be useful in data analysis (Krueger & Casey, 2000; Greenbaum, 2000). Different closing strategies can be used. A ranking strategy may be used, whereby participants are asked to rank all the issues discussed to identify those most important to them. For example, "Considering all the issues discussed this afternoon, which do you feel are the priority issues for government funding?" Alternatively, a summary strategy can be used, which involves the moderator giving a brief summary of the major issues discussed, then asking the group if this was an accurate reflection of the discussion. This ensures that important issues were not missed and allows participants to clarify points raised. Another closing strategy involves asking what message they would like to convey to a prominent person (e.g., a health minister, president, and policy-maker) about the issues discussed. For example, "Our discussion is almost over, but if you had just one minute with the Minister of Health what message would you like to convey from our discussion today?" This type of question can synthesize critical issues from the discussion and provides important perspectives on the issues discussed. It is worth allocating some time for the closing questions because they may elicit fruitful data or stimulate further discussion.

Question Design

The questions in a focus group discussion guide often seem deceptively simple, but in reality they are carefully designed to promote an effective group discussion. Although the question guide for a focus group discussion may seem similar to that used in an in-depth interview there are several key differences (Hennink, 2007). First, there are fewer questions in a focus group discussion guide because the questions are being asked of a group of people and there needs to be sufficient time for participants to respond and engage in a discussion. Second, questions for a focus group are phrased to promote a discussion rather than to elicit a single response, as in an in-depth interview. Third, questions are phrased to seek broad perspectives rather than personal narratives as is sought in an in-depth interview. Suggestions on designing questions for a focus group discussion are highlighted next.

Use clear, short, and simple questions. This ensures questions are easily understood and participants can respond. Questions need to sound informal and conversational to create a comfortable, non-threatening environment for discussion. Therefore, use colloquial language appropriate for the type of study participants and avoid technical jargon or academic language. In general, the longer the question the greater the loss of clarity; therefore, identify the shortest way to ask each question. Use simple questions, and remember that a simple question does not mean a simple answer will be given. Using clear, short, and simple questions also helps participants to remember the question as the discussion proceeds, therefore helping to keep the discussion focused on each issue.

Design open and uni-directional questions. Open questions allow participants to respond from any perspective allowing them to freely share their own views. For example, "What is your opinion of the new course on maritime law?" is an open question because it invites comments on any aspect of the course including positive and negative issues. Questions need to be uni-dimensional, asking about only one issue at a time. Avoid "double-barrelled" questions with multiple parts because participants may respond to different parts of the question causing a confused discussion. For example, "How does the cost and quality of the new facility compare with others in the neighbourhood?" is a double-barrelled question asking about cost and quality at once. Separating this into two short questions on cost and then quality is more effective.

Reduce dichotomous questions. A dichotomous question elicits a "yes/no" response and therefore does not promote discussion. At times a dichotomous question is needed to clarify whether partipants have certain knowledge or experience before asking more detailed questions on the topic. In this case follow the dichotomous question with an open question. For example, ask "Has anyone used the new aquatic centre?" (a dichotomous question) and then follow with an open question, such as "What were your first impressions of this facility?"

Avoid direct personal questions. The lack of confidentiality in a focus group means that personal questions can feel confrontational and make participants feel uncomfortable. Try to phrase questions in a less personal way. For example, rather than asking "Have you ever used drugs?" the same issue may be rephrased as "What type of drug use is common among your peers?" Participants may still respond with their own experience, but they choose to do so rather than feeling compelled by the wording of the question.

Design questions that promote discussion. Consider different questioning strategies that promote an interactive discussion. A useful strategy involves using a statement to promote a discussion. For example, by stating "We have heard people refer to this place as the 'poor people's clinic'. How do you think this affects clinic use?" This statement provides a tangible situation for participants to discuss. Similarly, using a vingette followed by a series of specifc questions can prompt a discussion of specific issues highlighted in the scenario.

Probes

The discussion guide usually includes questions followed by a series of probes (see examples in Figure 2.3). Probes are reminders for the moderator to ask about certain topics related to a question if they are not raised spontaneously by the group.

For example, the question below is followed by a series of probes:

Who is least likely to be able to pay for health insurance in this country?
(Probe: unemployed/low income, elderly, migrant workers).

A motivated group of participants may highlight a range of issues in response to a question. In the previous example participants may have spontaneously remarked that those who are unemployed, elderly, or have low income are least able to pay for health insurance; therefore, only the probes on insurance regarding migrant workers needs to be asked. Thus, not all probes are needed in every group discussion because many issues are raised spontaneously in response to the question, so the use of probes is guided by the discussion itself. Probes are used most often with the key questions in the discussion guide, because this is where the greatest depth of information is required. Probes initially originate from topics identified in a literature review. However, they are only indications of important issues to probe about, and they may be refined as data collection begins and more is learnt about what is important to the study participants themselves. In the previous example one may learn that students also face difficulties getting health insurance, so "students" may be added as a probe in subsequent group discussions.

Number of Questions

A discussion guide has a limited number of questions. It should be remembered that in a focus group discussion each question is being asked of a group of people, so there needs to be sufficient time for multiple participants to respond to each question, discuss the issue, and raise new issues. A single question in the discussion guide may therefore lead to 5–10 minutes of discussion or longer if the topic is controversial or participants have diverse views. Therefore, most discussion guides have 12–15 questions for a 1-hour discussion.

Having too many questions puts enormous pressure on the moderator to cover all questions in the discussion period, which may lead to superficial coverage of the issues and reduced data quality. It also provides no flexibility for the moderator to follow up on new issues raised or to fully probe the discussion for depth and detail. A focus group discussion is a dynamic activity and time is needed to fully explore the issues, for impromptu questions to be added, and for some deviation from the discussion guide to explore new issues raised. This flexibility is critical to the success of a focus group discussion and to qualitative research in general.

In addition, the topic of discussion and type of participants may influence the number of questions in the discussion guide. For example, a discussion among children or adolescents may include more questions because there may be less discussion than among a group of adults. Fewer questions may be included on a topic that is intense or emotional because more time may be spent discussing each issue. A discussion guide is typically designed for a group discussion of 1–2 hours. Longer sessions may lead to participant fatigue whereby the value of the information declines.

Data-Generating Activities

Conducting an activity in a focus group discussion can be an effective strategy to simultaneously build rapport, promote discussion, and generate data. An activity can immediately change a group dynamic, enabling participants to feel more at ease as they interact on a specific task. Therefore, activities can be effective in building rapport among participants. An activity can also effectively stimulate discussion. Even the simple task of ranking items in a list requires group interaction and discussion. In addition, an activity can provide an alternative means of collecting data on topics that may be difficult to discuss, by indirectly tapping into the thoughts and feelings of participants in a way that would otherwise be challenging through direct questioning. Therefore, an activity may elicit a different type of information that is complementary to the usual questioning strategies. One limitation of including an activity in a focus group discussion is that it reduces the time available for discussing other questions. Therefore, careful consideration of the value of an activity versus using simple questioning strategies is needed.

Many types of activities can be used in focus group discussions. Some activities involve writing, drawing, or responding to visual stimuli. For most activities the outcome of the activity provides data, such as the list developed, drawing created, or the verbal reactions to visual stimuli. However, where activities are intended to stimulate a discussion, it is often necessary to develop a set of questions related to the activity that tap into participants' thought processes and encourage them to critically reflect on issues raised by the activity. Therefore, many activities are followed by a set of discussion questions. When using activities, it is important to keep the focus group intact, rather than split participants into small groups. The intent of an activity is to promote discussion within the focus group itself, therefore creating small groups fragments the focus group and creates difficulties in recording multiple discussions, thereby losing valuable data.

When planning to use an activity in focus group research consider the following:

- What is the purpose of the activity?
- How will the activity promote interaction and discussion between participants?
- What type of data will be generated?
- How will the data be recorded (i.e., written or verbal)?
- What is the moderator's role during the activity?
- How do moderators need to be briefed?
- At what point in the discussion should the activity be conducted? (e.g., beginning or middle)
- How much time is needed for the activity?
- What equipment is needed (i.e., marker pens, cards, paper, and so forth)?
- Can the activity be piloted?
- How will including an activity affect other topics to be discussed?

A wide range of activities are commonly used in focus group discussions. Selecting an appropriate activity is determined by the study topic and overall purpose of the activity. Some activities and examples are given in the list below.

Types of Group Activities

Listing	Participants are asked to make a list of items, either individually or as a group. This can be followed up by ranking, comparing, or discussing items listed. For example, ask participants to collectively "Make a list of all the water sources in this village" or "List the benefits and limitations of the health screening program." Participants may make the list as a whole group or write individual lists and compare them in the discussion. Krueger and Casey (2009) caution against the moderator standing at a whiteboard to generate a list, because this can change the group dynamic with the moderator dominating the activity.

Ranking	Participants are asked to rank items by given criteria (e.g., cost, quality, effectiveness, convenience, and so forth). For example, a moderator may tell participants "Using the items on the list, rank them from the highest to lowest quality." They can be provided a pre-prepared list to rank or rank a list generated by the group itself.
Pile Sorts	Participants are asked to sort a range of images, photographs, or words into different piles by various criteria. They may be given criteria by the moderator or be asked to develop their own criteria of categories that distinguish items. For example, Quintiliani, Campbell, Haines, and Weber (2008) asked focus group participants to write down components of a healthy lifestyle (e.g., exercise, balanced diet, and so forth) on index cards and then sort these cards into piles according to their common characteristics. The piles were then discussed as a group guided by a moderator. In contrast, Kitzinger (1994, cited in Green & Thorogood, 2004) provided focus group participants with pre-prepared cards with statements about who was "at risk" from AIDS, which participants then sorted into groups of differing risk level. This activity prompted discussion among participants on the reasoning for the groupings, thereby providing valuable data on participants' assumptions and knowledge about AIDS. In addition, participants were provided a set of pictures from television and news reports and asked to construct a news report about AIDS.
Visual Props	Props are shown to the group to stimulate discussion, such as educational material (i.e., posters, video clips); current events (i.e., newspaper article, media clip); advertising material; and products. For example, in health research, props have included contraceptive devices, breast implants, and health promotion material, which are shown to the group for initial reactions followed by a series of questions for discussion.

Vignettes	A short scenario is read aloud to participants, followed by a series of specific questions. For example, participants may be asked what advice they would give to characters in the vignette, whether the scenario is common in their communities, how these issues are typically dealt with, and so on. Brondani et al (2008) describe using vignettes in focus group discussions with older adults to broach discussion on sensitive issues related to oral health. The vignettes included typical scenarios faced by older adults with dentures, which enabled participants to refer to situations in the vignette when discussing sensitive issues, such as personal hygiene, social expectations of facial appearance, and gender norms around oral hygiene.
Drawing	Participants are asked to make a drawing on a specific topic given by the moderator. Figure 2.4 shows a drawing developed in a discussion on stress among graduate students. Students were asked to draw a tree and then in the roots of the tree write all the causes of stress for graduate students. Examples in the drawing include "finances," "coursework," "thesis," "lack of sleep," and "future career." Students indicated that these stressors are compounded by time (as they depicted by the clock). They were then asked to write in the tree branches all the effects of stress. Some examples shown include "anxiety," "lack of exercise," "competitiveness," "exhaustion," and "isolation." After a drawing activity the moderator may lead a group discussion on the issues highlighted in the drawing, thereby providing valuable data that are inductively derived (from the drawing activity) and have depth and context (from the subsequent discussion).
Mapping	Participants are asked to sketch a map of their neighborhood and then mark certain items or places on the map as directed by the moderator. For example, participants may be asked to sketch a map of their neighborhood and then mark all the places they believe are safe or dangerous, hygienic or unhygienic, and so forth.

| Cartoons | Participants are asked to react to a cartoon or complete an empty speech bubble with a word or thought, which can effectively lead to a discussion. A cartoon may be used to begin a discussion on a difficult topic. Barbour (2007, p. 84) states that cartoons "often tap into and express succinctly in an amusing way, difficult and keenly felt dilemmas, but take the sting out of thinking about these. They thus, simultaneously break the ice and give permission to raise difficult issues." |

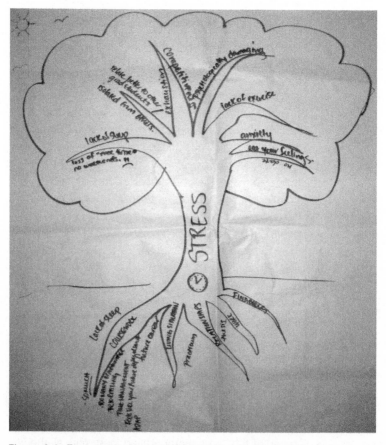

Figure 2.4. Example drawing activity depicting the root causes and outcome of stress.

Wherever possible it is important to pilot-test any stimulus material or activities to ensure they generate the intended type of discussion. For further reading on developing activity-oriented questions for focus group discussions see Colucci (2007). Many participatory tools, in particular community mapping, can also be effectively adapted for use in focus group discussions. For examples, see the selection of tools in International HIV/AIDS Alliance (2006).

Translating the discussion guide

When focus group discussions are conducted in a different language it is recommended to translate the discussion guide into the language of the discussion. Even when the moderator is bilingual a translated discussion guide is recommended. This takes a lot of pressure off the moderator who would otherwise need to translate each question spontaneously during the group discussion. This is described in an extract from a bi-lingual researcher in Zambia.

> I thought I am competent in the language of my country and I can read a question in English and directly translate it, no problem. But it proved very, very difficult. Translating it correctly from English to the local language, right there and then, was very, very difficult. The easier way is to translate the whole instrument into the local language and use the local languge. (Hennink, 2007, p. 66)

Translating the discussion guide allows the most appropriate colloquial language to be used so that questions are understood by participants as intended, thereby increasing data quality. Using appropriate colloquial language can also aid rapport development with participants. It is important that the translation uses an informal style of language appropriate to the study participants, because too formal language can create unwanted distance between the moderator and participants (Hennink et al., 2011). This type of translation can often be achieved by asking bilingual professionals from the study setting (i.e., teachers, nurses, and so forth) to translate the guide, rather than a professional translation service. It may be necessary to translate the discussion guide into several languages, particularly if the study is conducted in several regions of a country where different languages are used. In some countries there may be a national lingua franca that can be used.

The most important consideration is to identify the language in which participants would feel most comfortable to converse.

It is imperative to check the quality of the translation. Back-translation is a common strategy, whereby the text is translated back into the original language and checked for accuracy. What is most important is that the translation conveys the intended meaning of a question, rather than simply being an accurate translation of the words. Another strategy is to read translated questions to individuals familiar with the language and identify how each question is understood. For detailed guidance on translating a focus group discussion guide, selecting an appropriate language, and checking translations see Hennink (2007).

Piloting the discussion guide

It is good practice to pilot-test the discussion guide, because it can be difficult to predict how participants will interpret questions. Pilot-testing involves asking the discussion questions to a group of people with similar characteristics to the study population (if possible) or using the first focus group discussion as a pilot. After the pilot-test the questions and the overall structure of the discussion guide should be reviewed. Review questions to ensure they are clear, understood as intended, use appropriate language, are logically ordered, and there is no repetition or redundancy. Also, review the overall structure of the guide to assess the sequence of topics, number of questions, and the amount of time that participants discuss each issue. This may lead to reordering or removing questions to facilitate a smooth flow between topics and questions. The following questions (Hennink et al., 2011, p. 149) may be asked during the pilot-test:

- Was sufficient information given in the introduction to the group discussion?
- Were all questions understood as intended?
- Do any questions need to be re-worded to improve clarity?
- Is the structure of the discussion guide working well?
- Does the topic order need to change?
- Will the information help to answer the research question?
- Is the discussion guide an appropriate length for a 60–90 minute discussion?

The discussion guide is not a stand-alone instrument. The moderator is an important component in the delivery of questions and clarifications, and in probing the discussion. Therefore, the questions and their delivery by the moderator need to be assessed in the pilot-test. Pilot testing is thus an opportunity to also provide feedback to the moderator. During the pilot-testing it is important to identify whether any problem identified is caused by the design of the guide, the skills of the moderator, or perhaps issues related to the participant group. The guide can then be redesigned, the moderator retrained, or issues related to participants themselves can be reviewed.

Conducting Focus Group Discussions

Roles of Moderator and Note-Taker

Conducting the group discussion is the central activity in focus group research. It generates the study data; therefore, an effective group discussion is critical. Managing an effective discussion can be challenging and rewarding. A focus group discussion is typically conducted by a moderator and note-taker team.

A note-taker has multiple roles. Primarily they are responsible for writing down the key points raised in the discussion in as much detail as possible. The note-takers summary is important because it is the only record of the discussion if the recording device fails or participants refuse permission to record the discussion. The note-taker's summary needs to include the main points discussed and if possible key phrases or short sentences that reflect participants' expressions on critical issues. The summary should separate facts from any interpretation of the issues by a note-taker. In addition, a note-taker can also attend to any disturbances to the group, such as latecomers, so that the moderator can focus on conducting the group discussion. A note-taker sits outside the actual discussion circle to attend to these issues and to take notes unobtrusively. The note-taker can also operate the recording device and assist the moderator with other tasks that arise. More details on recording the group discussion are provided later in this chapter.

The moderator has the critical role of conducting the group discussion. In many ways the role of the moderator is similar to that of an interviewer in an in-depth interview in that they are responsible for developing rapport, collecting detailed data, pacing the session, and remaining focused on the research agenda. However, moderating a focus group discussion can be much more challenging because the moderator needs to manage a group of participants, which means greater skills and attention are needed in questioning and probing a whole group, fostering group cohesion, and managing the group dynamics, while remaining focused on the research objectives and facilitating the flow of an interactive discussion. Moderating a group discussion is a skilled activity, and the quality of the data generated depends on these skills. An experienced moderator uses a range of techniques to effectively manage the group discussion so that it yields useful information to meet the research objectives. These include adapting the level of moderation, effective listening, probing the discussion, seeking diverse views, or using activities to stimulate discussion. These techniques are discussed in the following sections. The moderator's roles are summarized next (adapted from Hennink et al., 2011, p. 155–166).

Provide Information
- Introduce the note-taker
- Describe the purpose of the study
- Outline how the group will be conducted (i.e., "guidelines")
- State the length of the discussion (e.g., 60 or 90 minutes)
- Answer participant's questions

Attend to Ethical Issues
- Indicate that participation is voluntary
- Confirm consent for participation
- Assure confidentiality of the discussion and data
- Ask permision to record the discussion

Enhance Group Cohesion
- Introduce all participants
- Create a comfortable, permissive environment
- Develop rapport with participants (e.g., friendly informal style)

Manage Group Dynamics
- Seek contributions from all participants
- Encourage quiet participants and manage dominant members
- Foster respect for different views

Facilitate the Discussion
- Encourage discussion between participants
- Seek a variety of views and experiences
- Use probing to seek depth and detail in responses
- Reflect positive body language to encourage discussion
- Listen to issues raised and follow leads for discussion
- Keep the discussion focused on research topics
- Determine whether responses provide sufficient information on each topic
- Invite new issues and opinions
- Vary moderation techniques to broaden or narrow the discussion
- Monitor timing and pacing of the discussion

The essential role of the moderator is to foster a productive group discussion that generates useful data to meet the research objectives. Managing a group discussion may seem straightforward but it involves a great deal of skill to facilitate the discussion and manage the group dynamics. A moderator's role involves building rapport with participants, which begins with creating a comfortable atmosphere and friendly tone in the introduction, in question delivery, and in encouraging participation. A moderator also needs to actively manage the discussion by carefully listening and following up participant's contributions; probing for depth, detail, and clarity; stimulating debate while fostering respect for diverse views; and courteously managing group dynamics. All these tasks need to be conducted similtaneously while focusing on the research objectives and intended outcomes of the study. The moderator also needs to pace the discussion, which not only involves covering all issues in the prescribed time period but also sensing when the group has exhausted one topic and is ready to move to the next.

The moderator must be familiar with the research objectives to make quick decisions during the discussion on whether new issues raised should be pursued or the discussion redirected back to topics in the guide. In many ways the moderator needs to remain focused and flexible.

The group moderator needs to ensure that the discussion remains focussed around the central research issues, yet allow sufficient divergence to identify new and unanticipated issues to emerge from the discussion. The moderator should encourage and manage a discussion, yet they should not dominate the discussion. The moderator needs to facilitate and channel the natural flow of the discussion, but not force it along a predetermined path. (Hennink, 2007, p. 177).

Although it is a moderator's imperative to ensure that the discussion remains focused on the research objectives, "in practice it can be difficult to decide when discussion goes off track, as participants may be developing a point that turns out to be germane, although this may not be clear from the outset" (Barbour, 2007, p. 106–107). Therefore, a moderator may often allow a group to continue to discuss a point until its relevance can be determined, whereby the moderator may either actively probe the issue or redirect the discussion. Furthermore, the moderator needs to be familiar with the questions on the discussion guide, the purpose of each question, and the approximate discussion time on each issue to effectively make decisions throughout the discussion process. Thereby, a moderator is continually thinking on their feet and making decisions on how to direct the discussion.

A key role of the moderator is to facilitate an interactive discussion among participants to achieve "non-directive interviewing" (described in Chapter 1). This provides the full benefit of using the focus group method. The core principle of non-directive interviewing is to move away from interviewer-dominated data collection and toward promoting a dynamic discussion among particiapants to access more spontaneous information than can be achieved through direct questioning. With this approach, the moderator's aim is to allow the discussion to emerge from the group itself while guiding it around the research topics. The group discussion format provides more scope for spontaneous issues to emerge than an individual interview, because there are multiple participants contributing to the discussion; the discussion becomes led more by the participants themselves with the moderator ensuring that key issues are covered in the allotted time (Ritchie & Lewis, 2003). Effective group interaction leads to participants essentially probing each other for explanations, justifications, clarifications, examples, or simply by entering into a dynamic discussion. When participants agree with one another this provides confirming data about an issue, whereas if they disagree the ensuing dialogue can provide greater insight into the differing perspectives of the issues, thereby providing greater depth and sponteneity to the resulting data. As Kitzinger states (1994, p. 107), achieving effective discussion between participants enables researchers to "reach parts that other methods cannot reach—revealing dimensions of understanding that often remain untapped by the more conventional on-to-one interview or questionnaire." Therefore, an interactive discussion can uncover new and unanticipated issues, which is a core goal of focus group research.

The style of moderation used can encourage or stifle discussion among participants. Figure 2.5 depicts a moderator-dominated discussion involving serial questioning of each participant versus an interactive discussion between participants with limited moderator involvement. A moderator should aim to acheive the latter dynamic, because a spontaneous discussion is less likely to occur with a more directive style of moderation (Hennink, 2007; Flick, 2002; Krueger, 1988). An effective focus group discussion is one where the moderator has limited input yet still subtly manages the discussion by probing participants, allowing time to explore issues, picking up on participants' cues, and keeping the discussion on the research issues. However, the moderator's level of direction may vary throughout the discussion, with a more directive style of moderation in the

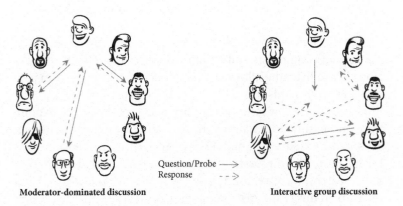

Question/Probe —→
Response - - →

Moderator-dominated discussion   Interactive group discussion

Figure 2.5. Types of group moderation. Adapted and reproduced with permission from Hennink, M., & Diamond, I. (1999). Using focus groups in social research. In A. Memnon & R. Bull (Eds.), *Handbook of the psychology of interviewing* (Chapter 2.5). Chichester, UK: Wiley & Sons.

beginning of the discussion to provide focus and a less directive approach during the central discussion to enable more sponteneous dialogue whereby new issues may emerge naturally.

When focus group discussions are conducted in another language, it may seem logical to conduct the discussion through an interpreter. However, an interpreter has a significant impact on the group dynamics and reduces the likelihood of creating an interative discussion, because each comment by a paticipant needs to be translated, which quickly stifles the flow of a natural discussion. A more effective strategy is to train a moderator fluent in the appropriate language to conduct the group discussion. See the earlier section on training a field team and also Hennink (2007) or Maynard-Tucker (2000) for further guidance on training moderators.

Active Listening

Listening is a key skill in effectively moderating a group discussion. Experienced moderators spend more time listening to participants than talking or questioning. Listening to participants' contributions allows the moderator to identify subtle cues in what is being said to redirect and manage the discussion without disrupting its momentum. When training a moderator "perhaps too much emphasis is placed on asking questions, when the real skill may be listening" (Barbour, 2007, p. 111). A moderator may use active and passive listening to moderate the discussion (Fern, 2001).

Active listening involves the moderator carefully listening to participant's comments and building on these to guide the discussion. Active listening allows the moderator to take cues from participants' comments to subtly direct the discussion. It allows the moderator to follow issues of importance to participants, explore these more fully, and maintain the natural flow of the discussion. This is the essence of qualitative interviewing. As the moderator listens to the discussion they are simultaneously considering the research objectives in deciding whether to follow the issues raised or redirect the discussion back to issues in the discussion guide. Therefore, it is an active task of listening, processing, and making decisions on how to guide the discussion. Active listening followed by effective probing (described later) are two basic moderation skills for facilitating an effective discussion.

A moderator may also use passive listening during the group discussion. Passive listening is a more empathetic task, whereby the moderator allows the discussion to flow naturally without interrupting or influencing the direction. "Knowing when not to intervene is, in itself, a skill...One of the hardest things for the novice moderator is perhaps taking a back seat and refraining from asking questions or making comments, provided that the discussion remains on track" (Barbour, 2007, p. 106). Passive listening may involve making positive and encouraging gestures to show interest in each contribution, but not direct the discussion as such. This approach is useful during a dynamic discussion to allow issues, responses, and dialogue to emerge naturally among participants. Thus, the moderator is essentially "leaning back" during parts of the discussion allowing the discussion to proceed uninterrupted. This strategy is most effective if used intermittently with active listening, whereby passive listening provides opportunities for participants to raise issues spontaneously thereby capturing new perspectives, and active listening provides direction to the discussion again.

Using Non-Verbal Cues

Using non-verbal cues given by participants can be an effective moderation strategy to encourage participation. Most moderators can feel participants' interest or enthusiasm for a topic that is independent of their actual contribution to the discussion (Fern, 2001). A moderator becomes familiar with certain facial expressions, gestures, or body language of participants that signal their desire to contribute to the discussion, disagreement with a speaker, or confusion about the dialogue. For example, frowning or shaking the head can indicate disagreement with what is being said; leaning back or looking away from the group may indicate boredom; whereas interest in the discussion may be signalled by attentiveness, leaning forward, and looking at a speaker. These non-verbal signals can be used to great effect by a moderator to stimulate further discussion or elicit views from individual participants. A moderator may notice one participant nodding as another speaks, and say, for example, "You are nodding, did you have a similar experience you would like to share with us?" Alternatively, a moderator may notice a participant frowning and simply ask "Do you disagree with this issue?" A moderator's attentiveness to non-verbal signals can dramatically increase participation in the discussion in a more natural way than calling on individuals at random for a contribution (Stewart & Shamdasani, 1990). A moderator needs to be aware, however, that although many non-verbal cues are universal some may have different meanings across cultures.

Motivational Probing

Motivational probes are short verbal cues used by the moderator to encourage participants to continue speaking. A motivational probe can be an encouraging word or phrase that is typically unspecific, for example uttering "uh-huh," "I see," or "ok" as a participant is speaking. This is different from topical probes written in the discussion guide (as described previously), which are specific topics related to a particular question (e.g., "cost" or "stigma") to remind the moderator to ask about this topic.

Motivational probes are very effective in gaining greater depth, clarity, and nuance on the issues discussed, which can greatly increase the quality and richness of the data. Motivational probing can also foster a positive group dynamic, because it indicates that the moderator is listening and interested in points raised by participants. Motivational probing is often used more at the beginning of the discussion to encourage participants to provide detailed contributions. However, one needs to take care not to overprobe participants, as this may stifle the discussion because participants may feel that the moderator is looking for specific responses.

A moderator can direct a motivational probe to an individual in the group in the same way as in an in-depth interview. The simplest example is uttering "uh-huh" to acknowledge a participant's contribution and encourage them to continue speaking. Other motivational probes for individuals include the reflective and expansive probes. The reflective probe involves the moderator paraphrasing a participant's comment for clarification and continued dialogue. The expansive probe seeks more information from a speaker by the moderator typically stating "Can you tell us more about that?" Additionally, the group format of a focus group provides a unique opportunity for a moderator to direct motivational probes to the whole group and thereby stimulate discussion. These group probes can be very effective in fostering interaction among participants and allowing a natural discussion to develop. Greenbaum (2000, p. 27) states that

> an important implied role of the facilitator is the ability to use moderation techniques that will 'peel away the onion' and delve into the real reasons for the attitudes or behaviours that are indicated. An integral part of this is to leverage the energy of the entire group to explore the topic area in depth.

A wide range of group probes can be used, as summarized below from Hennink et al. (2011, p. 162). Perhaps the most challenging is the silent probe. Silence can be very uncomfortable for a moderator. However, it is a simple and effective strategy that actually increases contributions to the discussion (Krueger & Casey, 2009). Conversely, too long a pause can have the opposite effect, therefore, a 5-second pause is typically recommended.

Types of Group Probes

Group probe	Seek further information from the group by using an issue raised by one participant to seek input from others. For example, "Jane raised an interesting point. Does anyone else have a similar experience?"
Group Explanation Probe	Ask the group to collectively explain an issue. For example, "Everyone seems to agree that the age of marriage should be 18 years. Can you all explain the reasons for this?" or "There seem to be several different views on the age of marriage, can you all explain the reasons for this difference?"
Ranking Probe	Ask the group to rank the issues raised, then provide reasons for their ranking. For example, "We have identified five problems in this community. Can you rank these in order of importance?" Then, "Why is this issue ranked first?"

Probe for Diversity	Ask for different views to seek diversity in opinions. For example, "Does anyone else have a different opinion or experience?" or "It seems like everybody has the same opinion, do you know whether others in the community have different views?"
Silent Probe	Remain silent for 5 seconds after a participant has spoken, to enable the speaker to expand their point or another participant to respond.

Managing Group Dynamics

One of the challenges of moderating a group discussion is managing the group dynamics. Every group has a range of personalities from those who are quiet to others who dominate the discussion. Kelleher (1982, cited in Krueger & Casey, 2009) estimates that 40% of participants are eager to share insights, another 40% are likely to be more introspective and contribute when the situation presents itself, and 20% are apprehensive and rarely share their views. A moderator's task is to manage the group dynamics that result from these personalities so that all participants have the opportunity to share their views. The moderator needs to be aware of how each of these personalities can affect group dynamics and use a range of strategies to manage each situation that arises. Some strategies are described next.

Quiet participants often remain silent during most of the discussion, providing only brief comments or responding only when called on. It can be easy to overlook a quiet participant, particularly when they are overshadowed by more dominant members. However, their opinions are equally important and it is the moderator's role to encourage their contribution. A quiet participant can often be encouraged to share their views with gentle probing by the moderator, open body language, and welcoming eye contact. A moderator may call on a quiet participant directly, but should be careful not to inhibit them by highlighting their silence. Inviting contributions that reinforce the value of their views can be most effective. For example, "Janice, we also value your views, do you have an opinion about this issue?" Reflect the value of their contribution by using it to stimulate a broader discusson, for example, "That's a good point what do others think?" Sometimes simply acknowledging the contribution of a quiet member is sufficient, for example, "Thank you. We have also heard this in other groups too." Participants who are quiet are likely to be acutely aware of their lack of engagement and the longer they remain silent the more difficult it may be to contribute. Therefore, gentle invitations to contribute by the moderator may come as welcome relief for these participants. Sometimes an entire group is quiet, and a moderator may need to take more time to develop rapport and reinforce the importance of participants' views. A quiet group may also be the result of poor participant selection, where a heirarchy has developed or participants feel they have little in common with others.

Many focus group discussions have a dominant participant who monopolizes the discussion. They may always be the first to respond to a question or to react to the comments of others, or provide lengthy or repetitive comments (Ritchie & Lewis, 2003). The challenge for the moderator is to allow a dominant participant to share their views but ensure that they do not overshadow others and inhibit their contributions. The moderator can use body language to signal reduced interest in the dominant participant once they have made their point, by reducing eye contact, turning a shoulder toward them, or looking down at the discussion guide. Occasionally, a moderator may need to use verbal cues to redirect the discussion away from the dominant member to allow other participants to contribute. For example, "Thank you for your views (then turn to the rest of the group). Perhaps we can hear the views of others as well?" or "Would anyone else like to comment on this point?" Usually a combination of verbal and nonverbal strategies begins to equalize contributions of group members. Moderators always need to remain tactful in these situations to avoid a negative impact on the group dynamic, and emphasize the importance of the dominant participant's comment before redirecting the discussion. If a moderator is ineffective in managing a dominant member, others in the group will begin to interrupt the dominant speaker to contribute their own views or they will simply lose interest and stop participating.

Some groups may include a rambling participant who feels very comfortable in the group and provides overly long responses or accounts that are of marginal or no relevance to the discussion issues. The moderator needs to manage a rambling participant because they take up the limited time for the group discussion and impede the ability for others to contribute in a similar way to a dominant participant. This may be achieved by reducing eye contact; redirecting the discussion (as described previously); or occasionally by interrupting them to enable others to contribute to the discussion.

Occasionally, a participant may proclaim that they are an expert on the topic with more knowledge than others in the group. These participants are rarely true experts, but they can easily create a hierarchy in the group whereby others begin to defer to them rather than share their own views. This situation can be particularly detrimental to group dynamics and quickly reduce the quality of the discussion. A moderator may disempower the "expert" by indicating that everyone in the group has expertise on the research topics, which is why they have been invited to the discussion, and that researchers are interested in the views of all group members. Occasionally, a participant has genuine expertise on the topic, whereby the moderator may acknowledge this but still emphasize that all perspectives are valued.

Some participants may have very strong views on the discussion issues, they may vehemently disagree with other views presented, or argue with other participants. A novice moderator may immediately try to quiet the argument or quickly move the discussion to the next topic to avoid conflict in the discussion. However, unless the argument was acrimonious and damaging to the group dynamics, then disagreement and thoughtful argument is a valuable contribution to the discussion, and a reminder to respect all participants points of view may be all that is needed. Barbour (2007, p. 81) offers the following advice, "focus groups allow the researcher to subtly set people off against each other and explore participants' differing opinions. Rather than seeking to move the discussion along...probe and invite participants to theorize as to why they hold such different views." This can result in fascinating insights on the different perspectives that adds valuable data to the study.

Group Location and Seating

A focus group discussion can be conducted in any type of location. They are often held in community settings, such as a town hall, school room, church, hotel, restaurant, offices, and in outdoor locations. An ideal location is quiet, private, comfortable, free of distractions, and easy to access.

A quiet location is critical for participants hear one another and to get a clear recording of the discussion. Always try to test the recording equipment at the location, because unexpected background noise may conceal participants voices making later transcription difficult. The location should be easily accessible for participants. Selecting a central community location or a venue regularly used by study participants is preferable. A neutral venue is also important. Sometimes materials at the venue (e.g., posters or advertising materials) can influence participants' contributions to the discussion. For example, a group discussion held at a health clinic displaying anti-abortion posters may influence how participants discuss this issue. Similarly, assess whether a venue has any particular associations for particpants. For example, a focus group held in the house of a prominent politician may lead participants to withold comments that do not align with that politician's views, even though they are not present at the discussion (Hennink et al., 2011).

Many focus group discussions are successfuly held outdoors. In some settings this is the only option available. Figure 2.6 shows a focus group discussion held outdoors. The main issue with

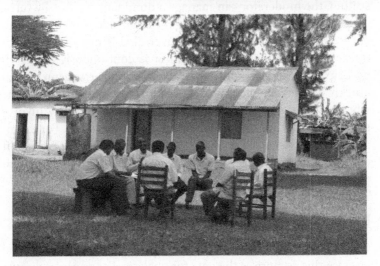

Photo: M. Hennink

Figure 2.6. Focus group discussion held outdoors in Uganda.

groups held outdoors is the lack of privacy. Participants may feel exposed or passers-by may stop to listen or join the group uninvited. Onlookers can disrupt group dynamics causing participants to withhold comments because of the lack of privacy. If onlookers join a group it may become too large and unweildly to moderate. These issues can be reduced by locating outdoor groups in a quieter part of the community, out of sight from pedestrian walkways or assigning an assistant to intercept and discourage onlookers from interrupting the group. For detailed guidance on effectively conducting outdoor focus group discussions see Hennink (2007).

Participants need to be seated in a circle, as shown in Figure 2.7 (panel 1). This is important for developing group rapport, facilitating group interaction, and managing the discussion. Vaughn, Shay, Schumm, and Sinagub (1996) state that participants communicate most with those seated directly across from them. Therefore, circular seating enables participants to have eye contact with others in the group, which fosters interaction. A linear seating arrangement (as shown in Figure 2.7, panel 2) hampers eye contact among participants, which is counterproductive for group interaction and discussion. A linear arrangement may quickly become a moderator-dominated session, or result in participants anticipating a presentation by the moderator. Circular seating also aids in effectively managing the group discussion. With circular seating, the moderator can manage a dominant speaker by turning a shoulder toward them, facing the other side of the circle, and encouraging other speakers. However, this is not possible with linear seating because the moderator is continuously facing all participants and cannot turn away. Poor seating arrangements can quickly hamper an effective discussion. Therefore, select a venue where seating can be arranged appropriately. This may involve some improvization with what is available at the venue. For example, benches were used in Figure 2.7 (panel 1) to form a makeshift circle. In outdoor groups, mats may be placed on the ground and participants asked to sit in a circle.

Recording the Discussion

Obtaining an accurate record of the group discussion is critical because this comprises the data for analysis. Focus group discussions are typically recorded in two ways: with an audio recorder

Panel 1: Circular seating

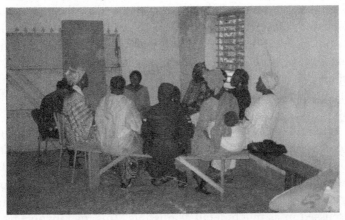

Panel 2: Linear seating

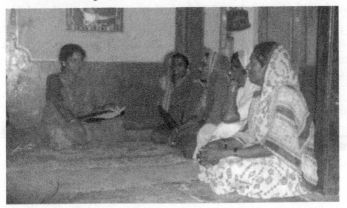

Photo: M. Hennink

Figure 2.7. Seating of focus group participants (Panels 1 and 2).

and a note-taker's written summary. Audio recording is preferred because it offers a verbatim record of the discussion, which is necessary for some approaches to data analysis, such as grounded theory. However, not all participants may consent to audio record the discussion; therefore, note-taking remains an important backup.

Note-Taking

A note-taker is part of the focus group team, who attends the group discussion to develop a written summary of the key issues raised (see the previous section on a note-taker's role). The note-taker's summary should focus on recording the main points discussed, rather than interpretation or judgment about what is said. In addition, a note-taker may record participants' body language, or note whether the discussion was lively, heated, or subdued around specific issues. This can add insight to the issues during data analysis, but is not mandatory and can be somewhat subjective.

A note-taker's role is critical because they are generating data; therefore, they need to be throughly briefed before the task. It is not possible to write down everything said in a fast-paced discussion. A note-taker's summary should therefore aim to reconstruct the main flow of the discussion, highlighting key issues discussed in as much detail as possible. This may involve paraphrasing discussion points, and noting some phrases or comments verbatim that exemplify critical issues raised. A note-taker typically writes notes in the same language as the discussion itself. This enables them to focus on the discussion and capture key phrases verbatim. If necessary, the notes can be translated after this discussion.

A note-taker's summary should be clearly labelled and structured. Each written summary may be labelled with key characteristics about the group, such as the date; start and end time of the discussion; number of participants; participant characteristics (e.g., women younger than 30 years); name of moderator and note-taker; location of the discussion; and any other information relevant to the project. A clear structure is also important. Using a template may help a note-taker to structure their notes during the discussion. For example, using a three-column table, whereby the first column lists each question in the discussion guide, the second column summarizes participants' responses to each question, and a third column may be used for a note-taker's additional comments. Similarly, Krueger and Casey (2009) recommend a two-column table for summarizing "notes" and "quotes," with a horizontal line separating each question or topic discussed. Using a template can be very effective for a structured discussion, but less effective for a more free-flowing discussion where a note-taker may become frustrated on where to include comments that are not clearly aligned with a question on the template. Therefore, taking notes freely (without a template) can be equally as effective at capturing the flow of a discussion. Whichever method is used a note-taker's summary should be written in full within 24 hours of the discussion and certainly before the next group discussion so as not to confuse the issues raised in each group.

Audio- and Video-Recording

A focus group discussion is typically recorded using an audio-recording device. Audio-recording provides an accurate, verbatim record of the discussion, which enables researchers to use quotations of participants' own words when reporting issues discussed. This is a tradition of qualitative research. Participants' permission should always be sought before audio-recording the discussion. Taking time to explain the purpose of recording the discussion and how it will be used and safeguarded often dispels participant concerns about using the recorder (Hennink, 2007). However, if permission is refused, the note-taker's summary becomes the only record of the discussion (described previously).

The recording device is placed in the center of the discussion circle and is typically operated by the note-taker. It is good practice to test the audio-recorder at the venue for any interference that may reduce the quality of the recording, and to carry replacement batteries. There are many affordable, high-quality digital recorders now available, which provide high-quality sound, have large memory storage, and a USB connection to immediately download the recording.

Video-recording of focus group discussions is not common in social science research. There is often little reason to capture a visual record of the discussion in addition to the audio-recording. Although video can capture participants' body language and facial expressions, many researchers remain concerned about the intrusiveness of video-recording. The presence of a video-recorder can influence participants' contributions to the discussion and thereby reduce data quality. For this reason, the benefits of video-recording need to be balanced against the potential impact on participants' contributions. The purpose of obtaining a visual record of the discussion needs to be made clear to participants, and their consent is always required.

Using Court Reporters

Some researchers are beginning to use court reporters to capture a "real-time" record of a focus group discussion (see for example, Jennings, Loan, Heiner, Hemman, & Swanson, 2005; Newhouse, 2005; Kick, Adams, & O'Brien-Gonzales, 2000). Court reporters are trained transcriptionists who are used to create a verbatim record of court proceedings, but can also be used to record meetings or closed-caption media steaming.

A court reporter may be used to create a verbatim record of a focus group discussion. The court reporter is present at the focus group discussion and simultaneously listens to the discussion and types into a stenotype machine using specialized shorthand. This is then transformed into a verbatim transcript in real-time. The benefits of using a court reporter include the immediacy of the written transcript (Scott et al., 2009); potential for greater accuracy (Easton, McComish, & Greenberg, 2000); and because court reporters are present at the group discussion, they can also note body language and identify speakers on the transcript. This method of recording a focus group discussion eliminates any problems associated with audio equipment or poor-quality recording. Despite the appeal of using a court reporter there are some drawbacks. In a formal evaluation of court reporters and transcriptionists for qualitative research, Hennink and Weber (2013) reported that court reporters were actually shown to make more errors in transcription, particularly in the topical content of the discussion, and were less able to produce a verbatim transcript with colloquial dialogue. However, the potential immediacy of the transcript was advantageous. The cost of court reporters varied but they were found to be more cost effective than transcriptionists for longer focus group discussions (Hennink & Weber, 2013). Understanding the benefits and drawbacks of court reporters is therefore necessary if selecting this method of recording focus group discussions.

Analyzing Focus Group Data

The systematic analysis of focus group data is what distinguishes the academic approach to focus group research from the market research approach (Bloor et al., 2001). Focus group discussions produce textual data that can be analyzed using a range of analytic approaches. The method of analysis selected depends on the purpose of the study. For example, focus group research may be conducted to inform the development of a quantitative survey; therefore, intense in-depth analysis may not be required. Other studies use focus group data to understand social processes or explain behavioral norms for which more extensive analysis and theory building is needed. Therefore, the approach to analyzing focus group data varies from study to study. The analytic strategy used is guided by the purpose of the study, how the study outcomes will be used, and the resources available for analysis.

Many analytic approaches require data to be transcribed to produce a written record of the discussion for analysis. Transcription requirements are influenced by the analytic approach selected. For example, thematic analysis, grounded theory, and discourse analysis require a verbatim transcript. Conversation analysis has additional transcription requirements, because the purpose is to analyse how participants express themselves; therefore, the transcription needs to include detail on word emphasis, pronunciation, elongation of words, hesitations, the length of pauses, and so forth.

Approaches to Analyzing Focus Group Data

It is worthwhile to note that "focus groups are distinctive...primarily for the method of data *collection* (i.e. informal group discussion), rather than for the method of data analysis" (Wilkinson, 2011, p. 169). Therefore, focus group data are typically analyzed using conventional methods of qualitative data analysis. Three main approaches are commonly used to analyze focus group data: (1) qualitative content analysis; (2) thematic analysis; and (3) constructionist methods (e.g., discourse analysis, conversation analysis). Perhaps the most common of these is thematic analysis or variations on this approach.

Approaches to data analysis can broadly be divided into those that break-up data into segments or themes for analysis (e.g., content analysis, thematic analysis) and those that do not break-up data but analyze the whole narrative (e.g., discourse analysis, conversation analysis). Even within this categorization there is variation in the analytic strategies used. For example, even though content analysis and thematic analysis involve breaking data into defined parts, their analytic approach is quite different. Content analysis essentially involves counting defined items in the data and generating frequency counts of each item. This produces a distribution of items across the data set but loses the descriptive context of how participants describe issues. Thematic analysis also involves breaking-up data by substantive themes, but instead of counting these themes per se (as in content analysis) it provides a descriptive account of the issues using illustrative quotations to highlight issues in participants' own words. Therefore, both these approaches take the unit of analysis as the mention of an issue, but each records these mentions differently—content analysis records the *number* of mentions, whereas thematic analysis records the *words* and context in which these mentions are described (Wilkinson, 2011). Therefore, there exist distinctly different approaches to analysis of textual data.

Other approaches to analysis consider the whole narrative in context, rather than breaking-up data. In constructionist methods, for example, the unit of analysis is broader than individual contributions to a discussion and includes whole discussions or narratives. In this approach, the outcome of analysis reports how issues are constructed in the discussion; the sequence of talk; and the interactive component of the dialogue, which influences the social construction of meaning in a group discussion. Parker and Tritter (2006, p. 34) state that "attention must be paid to the dynamic aspects of interaction within the group, for it is this dynamic nature which is at the heart of focus groups and which endow them with the power to generate insight often negated by other methods." Constructionist approaches can be useful when identifying a group narrative on the issues and how this narrative was constructed.

These approaches to analyzing focus group data are outlined next. It is not the intention here to provide a "how to" guide for analysis of focus group data, but rather to indicate various analytic approaches for readers to further explore independently.

Qualitative Content Analysis

Qualitative content analysis is a classic approach for analyzing textual data (e.g., media documents; records; speeches; narrative data, such as interviews) or visual data (e.g., posters, photographs, videos). It is a systematic approach to counting and categorizing specific items in data to identify their frequency and patterning.

Content analysis involves "examination of the data for instances of some kind; these instances are then systematically identified across the data set" (Wilkinson, 2011, p. 170). These may be instances of words, phrases, discourses, or other identifiable occurrences, which are marked in the transcript by a coding system and then tabulated across the data as a whole to produce basic frequency counts. The focus of content analysis is therefore to identify how often specific things are mentioned and to identify any patterns in these occurrences. Content analysis involves the quantification of items in qualitative data. This provides a sense of the overall distribution of each item across the data as a whole. Bernard and Ryan (2010) distinguish seven basic steps to conducting qualitative content analysis:

1. Formulate a research question to apply to data
2. Select a set of texts (or other data) to analyze
3. Create a set of codes that define items to observe in data (e.g., words, phrases)
4. Pretest the codes
5. Apply codes to data where items are observed
6. Create a case by variable matrix of the frequency of occurrence of each item
7. Analyze the matrix using whichever level of analysis is appropriate

Qualitative content analysis can be used to identify the frequency of certain words in data. For example, how often do participants mention the word "stress"; does the frequency of "stress" differ between focus groups with different types of participants (e.g., employed vs. unemployed participants). Tools for content analysis include searching "key words"; "key-word-in context"; word frequency counts; and space measurement tools (e.g., measuring lines of text on stress). Software is available with these tools. A further refined application of qualitative content analysis is to identify a range of items for the coding frame inductively (from a prior thematic analysis of the text) and then tabulate the frequency that each item is mentioned. For example, in a study on the causes of breast cancer, researchers identified 12 causes of breast cancer that were mentioned by focus group participants and then conducted a frequency count on the number of instances each cause was mentioned in the data (Wilkinson, 2011). This differs from thematic analysis (described next) in that the causes of breast cancer are counted in content analysis, rather than examining participants' experiences as in thematic analysis.

For further reference on the use of qualitative content analysis see Bernard and Ryan (2010), Denzin and Lincoln (2008), Grbich (2007), Krippendorf (2004), and Weber (1990).

Thematic Analysis

Thematic analysis is perhaps the most common approach to analyzing focus group data. It involves breaking data into smaller segments by using the issues raised by participants to define the segments. It is an inductive approach to analysis that involves immersion in the data. This allows each issue to be analyzed in depth and the relationships between issues to be identified, to build an understanding of the research issues from the perspective of study participants. This analytic process can build evidence-based descriptions or explanations about social phenomenon leading to the development of sociological theory. Thematic analysis requires a verbatim transcript of the group discussion, so that participants' own expressions and perspectives can be identified. One of the hallmarks of thematic analysis is the use of quotations to illustrate specific issues in participants' own words.

One of the challenges of thematic analysis for focus group data is that segmenting data takes away the interactive narrative within which issues are embedded. The focus of analysis is on issues raised by individuals, with little attention on the group context within which an individual's comments are made, and which may influence the issues raised. Given the value placed on group interaction in generating focus group data, removing this context when analyzing data and not acknowledging group interaction can seem counter to the nature of the data itself (Wilkinson, 2011; Kitzinger, 1994).

Thematic analysis encompasses several analytic approaches, the most notable of which is grounded theory. Many researchers use variants of the classic grounded theory approach. Grounded theory is a prominent approach for qualitative data collection and analysis. Its initial development (Glaser & Strauss,

1967) and its subsequent variations (Charmaz, 2006; Strauss & Corbin, 1998) have remained influential in qualitative research for the past four decades. Grounded theory provides a flexible set of guidelines and a process for analyzing textual data toward the development of empirical theory. It can be used for analyzing any form of textual data, including focus group discussions. The process of analysis begins with developing a verbatim transcript, then identifying a core set of themes that are raised in the discussion. Data are then systematically indexed (or coded) by each theme so that all comments around a single issue can be retrieved and reviewed in detail. Analysis often begins with developing descriptive accounts of central themes in the data. A detailed description of the core themes provides the foundation for analysis and gives the depth, richness, and nuances that are characteristic of qualitative analyses. Comparison is a core task in grounded theory, whereby themes may be compared across the data to identify patterns, for example comparing differences between focus groups with men and women on particular issues. Themes may also be categorized leading to a higher level of abstraction from the data toward empirical theory-building to explain or understand the social phenomenon studied. Grounded theory also offers numerous techniques to verify that the theory or explanations developed are well grounded in the empirical data. The results of grounded theory analysis may be illustrated with quotations from the data or presented in the form of an empirical conceptual framework.

Wilkinson (2011) provides a useful comparison of using thematic analysis and content analysis to highlight the differing approaches and analytic outcomes. For further guidance on thematic analysis, see Guest, MacQueen, and Namey (2012); for grounded theory and its variants, see Glaser and Strauss (1967), Strauss and Corbin (1998), and Charmaz (2006).

Constructionist Approaches

Constructionist approaches seek to understand the conversational character of data by examining how meanings are constructed through interactive dialogue. Common analytic methods that use the constructionist approach include narrative analysis, discourse analysis, and conversation analysis.

In constructionist approaches, the narrative flow of the data is kept intact so that the sequence of talk can be assessed, rather than segmenting data as in the other analytic approaches described previously. In focus group data, interactions among group participants and between the moderator and participants are examined. The main focus of analysis is on identifying a broad discourse or group narrative that is produced from the discussion. The purpose of constructionist approaches is to identify the social construction of meaning that occurs through an interactive dialogue (Silverman, 2011a), rather than focusing on individual contributions to the discussion. These approaches provide a unique opportunity to observe participants' understanding of issues, how they present issues through dialogue, or how the dialogue itself shapes perspectives. Researchers wishing to examine collective identity can capitalize on the opportunity these approaches offer to analyze the formation of a group narrative and to capture the narrative itself (Liamputtong, 2011; Munday, 2006).

Although the main focus of constructionist methods is on conversational structure, Silverman (2011a) describes that this approach can also provide valuable insights on the substance of the issues discussed. He uses the example of a study by Wilkinson (2011) that used a constructionist approach to identify perceptions on the causes of breast cancer. Analysis involved examining the sequence of dialogue among participants, the nature of their interaction, and the positioning of the speakers in the narrative. This analysis identified how participants used interactional devices, such as how speakers presented beliefs on the causes of breast cancer as "stories" related to them by others not as their own beliefs; how some potential causes of breast cancer were voiced by participants and then withdrawn; and how a possible lack of knowledge about causes of breast cancer may be averted in conversational dialogue. This type of analysis provides fascinating insight into the construction of meaning through conversational structures. In addition, the same data provided a broader group narrative about how "positive thinking" is a socially constructed expectation assumed to assist people to cope better with cancer; yet participants' actual internal responses to becoming diagnosed were fear and sadness (not positive thinking). In contrast, a thematic analysis may have identified segments of text on "positive thinking" as a theme in the data. However, the constructionist approach analyzed how participants talked about positive thinking to reveal a dual narrative on the expected societal response versus the actual personal response to their diagnosis. Constructionist approaches can therefore provide insights on substantive issues by analyzing the way in which people talk in a group discussion, to uncover underlying narratives or understandings that would be masked by other analytic approaches that segment data.

For further information on using constructionist methods see Grbich (2007), Rapley (2007), Elliott (2005), and Phillips and Hardy (2002). For a detailed comparison of constructionist methods and content analysis see Wilkinson (2011) and Silverman (2011a).

Key Points

....

- Focus group research requires careful planning, design, and training of the field team.
- A focus group discussion typically includes six to eight participants to provide diversity in views yet remain manegable for the moderator.
- Two aspects of group composition are important: homogeneity of participants and their level of acquaintance.
- Qualitative research uses purposive (non-random) recruitment of participants, because the aim is not to generalize findings to a broader population but to gain a detailed contextual understanding of the study issues.
- Ethical issues need to be assessed throughout the research process, because of the continually evolving nature of data collection and the group context in which data are collected.
- A discussion guide is a prepared list of topics or questions used by the moderator to guide the group discussion. It often follows an hourglass design moving from broad to specific questions and back to broad questions.
- A discussion guide usually includes 12–15 questions, including an introduction, opening question, introductory questions, key questions, and closing questions. Activities are sometimes included.

- A focus group is conducted by a moderator and note-taker team. The moderator facilitates the group discussion, whereas the note-taker records key issues raised.
- A skilled moderator is needed to facilitate the discussion, manage group dynamics, and effectively probe participants to generate useable data.
- Focus group discussions are typically recorded in two ways: by an audio-recorder and a note-taker.
- Common approaches to analyze focus group data include qualitative content analysis; thematic analysis; and constructionist methods (e.g., discourse analysis, conversation analysis).

3

WRITING FOCUS GROUP METHODS

THE RESEARCH METHODS section is a critical component of any research report. Not only does the methods section need to provide the procedural detail of how the study was conducted, it also provides context to the study and is used to assess the quality of the research. Writing the methods section of a focus group study may present some challenges in effectively describing and justifying the methodological procedures used and in determining how to effectively demonstrate scientific rigor throughout the research process to show that the study results are valid.

This chapter begins with a description of the challenges in writing the methods section of a focus group report. Many of these challenges apply to writing qualitative methods in general, not only the focus group method. It then describes the purpose and content of the methods section. Guidance is provided on what to include in the methods section, why each component is important, and suggestions on how to write each part. Examples of extracts from published focus group research are used throughout the chapter to demonstrate how particular aspects of the methods section can be written. Common pitfalls in writing the methods section are described, as is how to overcome these pitfalls.

The next chapter discusses how to write the results section of focus group research. The focus of this book, on writing the methods and results sections of focus group research, is warranted because they are central components to any research report and often present the greatest writing challenges for qualitative researchers. The emphasis of both chapters is on writing for academic audiences.

Challenges of Writing Focus Group Methods

Writing research methods can be challenging because of the multiple roles of this part of the research report. The methods section needs to simultaneously report procedural detail, provide scientific justifications, and reflect methodological rigor. In addition, the methods section needs to identify qualitative concepts and procedures used, but also explain them to readers unfamiliar with specific terminology. The methods section also needs to effectively reflect the context of the study, which influences the study outcomes. Overall, the methods section needs to provide methodological depth yet be written concisely, and present a logical process from what is a more circular iterative research approach. These challenges are briefly highlighted next and are reflected throughout this chapter.

Procedural Detail

There is no single way to conduct qualitative research or focus group discussions. Therefore, in writing the research methods the challenge lies in providing sufficient transparency on how focus groups were conducted and the methodological decisions that shaped the study process. The methods section needs to describe both the procedural detail and scientific reasoning to demonstrate the rigor of the study. Therefore, a reader should be clear on both what was done and why it was done in that way.

In addition, the overall process should be clear, by describing each step undertaken in a logical progression. There should be sufficient detail for another researcher to (potentially) repeat the tasks and follow the logic of decisions made. Too often there are gaps in the description of qualitative research methods, leaving a reader unclear on what was done at a certain stage of the research process. This is particularly true in the description of data analysis, whereby data preparation is often described in detail (e.g., transcription, code development, coding of data, intercoder assessment), but then little or no description is provided on how the data were subsequently analyzed after these components of data preparation. For example, were analytic tasks used, such as description or comparison; how were concepts developed; how was a conceptual framework or theory developed and validated; and so on. Similarly, descriptions of participant recruitment are often incomplete, naming only a strategy without describing how it was applied in the study context. The methods section therefore needs to be logical, comprehensive, and detailed. An effective way to assess if all necessary detail is included in a methods section is to ask another researcher to read and subsequently describe in their own words what was done and why; this can uncover gaps in the process or unclear reasoning.

Writing Concisely

A further challenge of writing focus group research is to write concisely yet provide the necessary procedural detail and methodological justifications that give the study scientific credibility. This is particularly challenging when writing within the word limits imposed by academic journals. The methods section of a qualitative report is often longer than for other types of research. In part, this is because of the non-standard application of qualitative methods, which requires a more detailed description of the research strategy and justifications for methodological decisions and procedures used. "Qualitative researchers employ less standardised data collection methods, ways of developing analytic categories and modes of organising evidence. The methods chosen depend on the conditions of the research site and the researchers' preferences. Hence, qualitative research needs to explain what, and why, they did what they did in greater detail" (Liamputtong & Ezzy, 2007, p. 309). This need to explain and justify the research procedures adds length to a methods section. In addition, the credibility of the study is assessed through the rigor of the methodological approach applied; therefore, sufficient detail needs to be presented. Although adding length to the methods section this detail is critical.

Reflecting the Interpretive Approach

Focus group discussions are a method of qualitative research. Therefore, writing the research methods needs to reflect the interpretive paradigm within which the research was conducted. This relates to describing the process of data collection and analysis, referring to appropriate techniques and concepts, and using relevant terminology. When describing the research process, refer to the circular, iterative nature of qualitative data collection and how this was operationalized in the study. The iterative process is not only a hallmark of qualitative data collection but also provides an indicator of quality data collection. In describing data collection and analysis, refer to methodological concepts that are relevant to the interpretive paradigm and describe how these were applied to the study. For example, refer to *purposive* (non-random) recruitment of participants; state how *saturation* (the point where no new information is gained) was used to determine an appropriate number of participants; refer to the *emic* perspective (participants' viewpoint) and how this was obtained in the study; and describe how *reflexivity* (assessing a researcher's subjective influence on the study) was used through the study. These concepts and terminology situate the study clearly within the interpretive paradigm.

Although it is important to use terminology appropriate to the interpretive paradigm, such terminology should not be used without briefly indicating what the concept is and how it was specifically applied to the study. Belgrave, Zablotsky, and Guadagno (2002) caution to "use technical language, but don't use it alone" (p. 1431), because not all readers are familiar with qualitative research and the methodological concepts it embraces, or there may be variations in how certain concepts are understood. It is better to "waste" space to explain a concept to readers than to have them misunderstand what was actually done. Therefore, the challenge is to report focus group research within the parameters of the interpretive paradigm to reflect scientific rigor, and to use relevant methodological terminology to do so, but also embrace readers who may not be familiar with the terminology or concepts used. Furthermore, it is important not only to mention particular concepts, but to describe how they were applied to the specific study. Avoid providing a generic description of focus group research or using terminology to provide methodological "labels" in the methods section. For example, rather than stating "purposive recruitment was conducted," "grounded theory was used," or "saturation was achieved," describe exactly how this was done in the context of the study. This inevitably requires providing specific methodological detail that reflects the study purpose, context of the study, or particular methodological challenges. These details provide specificity to the research methods section and allow the opportunity to justify methodological decisions and procedures.

Reporting Context

Examining the context of social issues is a well-known characteristic of qualitative research and may be the explicit purpose of a focus group study. These contextual influences form part of the study findings and are therefore reported in the results section of the research report. However, contextual issues also influence data collection in qualitative research, but reporting this aspect of context is often overlooked when writing the research methods. There are various types of context that can be described in the methods section. For example, the theoretical context of the study phenomenon underlies the research question and the development of research instruments, and can be reflected when describing the topics or questioning strategies used in the focus group discussions. The socio-cultural context of the study site is perhaps the most tangible aspect of context included in the research methods. This may include a description of broad social issues and cultural behaviors that may impact on the research topic. The methodological context of data collection refers to describing the study design and the context in which focus group discussions were conducted. This may include describing the physical setting where focus groups were conducted and the group context of data collection. Finally, a brief description of the broader sociopolitical context in which the study was conducted is warranted because this constitutes the political, administrative, or governance structures and boundaries within which the study recommendations need to be shaped. All these aspects of context influence the study design, implementation, and outcomes. They help the reader to understand contextual influences that shaped each stage of the study and provide the backdrop against which the study results need to be interpreted.

Demonstrating Rigor

A critical role of the methods section is to demonstrate scientific rigor and reflect research quality. This adds a critical dimension to writing qualitative research methods that is often overlooked. There is no single way to conduct a focus group study, therefore, it is imperative not only to describe the study procedures but also the justifications and reasoning for methodological choices. Describing what was done (research tasks), how it was done (methodological procedures), and why it was done this way (scientific reasoning) demonstrates rigor in the research process. A further reflection of rigor involves appropriately referring to procedures, concepts, and terminology relevant to the interpretive paradigm within which focus group research is conducted (as described previously). The research methods section is central to determining the rigor and crediblity of the study; therefore, providing procedural detail needs to be balanced with methodolgic justifications. Strategies for conducting rigorous focus group research are described in Chapter 2, and reflecting research quality is described in Chapter 5.

Writing the Methods Section

Purpose of the Methods Section

The methods section of a research report has multiple functions: it simultaneously needs to describe the research process, set the context of the study, and reflect the quality of the research. Therefore, the methods section is a critical component of any research report. It is important to understand these multiple functions because they indicate how the methods section is read and assessed by different types of readers.

A basic function of the methods section is to describe the research process. It needs to tell the reader what was actually done, how it was done, and why it was done this way. Therefore, the methods section needs not only to identify each step in the research process and describe how it was implemented, but it also needs to provide a rationale for the methodological decisions made. Given that there is not one single formula for conducting focus group research and researchers may need to navigate certain fieldwork constraints, the methods section needs to provide an insight into the decisions that shaped the research process and its outcomes. A methods section needs to provide the most comprehensive description possible within the word limit available. This may involve presenting some information in visual format (e.g., tables or figures). An effective methods section provides the reader with sufficient procedural information to enable them to repeat the research process and understand the methodological decisions made.

The methods section also needs to provide context to the study. It is not only important to describe the socio-cultural context in which the study was conducted, but also the methodological context in which data were collected. Providing methodological details about the nature of focus group research and how group discussions were conducted enables readers to correctly interpret the study findings and understand the purpose and limitations of this type of data. Furthermore, the context of the research design is also important. Whether focus group discussions were the core method used or if they supplemented other methods in the study provides important contextual information on the role of focus groups within the larger context of the study.

A third function of the methods section is to demonstrate research quality. The flexible nature of qualitative research means that it is not conducted in a standardized way. Therefore, there is a greater need than for other types of research to describe the procedural steps and methodological decisions that demonstrate scientific rigor. The methods section is thus an opportunity for researchers to demonstrate the quality of the study by providing a transparent description of the research process undertaken and the methodological decisions and challenges that influenced the study outcomes. Although the quality of a study is demonstrated throughout a research report, the methods section provides the procedural details on data collection and analysis from which to judge the credibility of the study findings. Therefore, the methods section has a critical role in allowing readers to assess the scientific rigor of the study and overall research quality (see Chapter 5 for discussion on assessing quality).

The Target Audience

A basic rule of writing is to consider the target audience, because this influences all aspects of writing. The target audience determines the structure, content, language, style, and length of the methods section. Even though the primary audience may be academics, there may also be a need to present the study to other audiences, such as policy makers, practitioners, advocacy groups, community members, non-goverment organizations, or media sources. Therefore, several versions of the methods section may be needed to suit different audiences.

Academic audiences (more than others) expect the methods section to be embedded in a theoretical framework that reflects the scientific literature on the topic, use appropriate methodological terminology, and describe measures that reflect scientific rigor. The theoretical or conceptual framework of the study is generally described in earier sections of the report. The methods section needs to reflect the theoretical framework of the study by demonstrating how the study design, research question, and research methods operationalize the broader theoretical framework of the study. For example, the theoretical framework may be referred to when describing the selection of topics or questioning strategies used in the focus group discussion guide, the rationale for the types of participants recruited, or the analytic approach selected. Embedding the research methods within a broader theoretical framework reflects the scientific rigor expected of academic audiences. In addition, refering to appropriate research techniques and using methodological terminology and academic language are additional features of writing for academic audiences. These components often mean that the methods section of an academic report is longer than for other types of audiences.

Although the previously mentioned components are expected in an academic report, academic audiences come from diverse disciplines and have varying experience of qualitative research. Not all readers are familiar with qualitative research or focus group discussions, how they are conducted and why, the type of evidence produced, and what they can and cannot do. Therefore, in addition to tailoring the research methods section to a specific type of audience, it also needs to be understood more broadly, in particular by those less familar with focus group research. This is not to say that methodological terminology should be avoided, but that it may need to be explained so that all readers can follow the logic of procedures described.

Non-academic audiences, such as policy makers or nongovernment agencies, have different requirements and expectations of the research report. They typically place less emphasis on the theoretical and methodological components of the study, instead giving prominence to key findings and implications for policy and practice. Writing for these audiences is typically shorter, little academic terminology is used, the study findings are highlighted and are often placed first, and research methods are often de-emphasized. Therefore, the first task in writing focus group research is to identify the target audiences and understand their requirements.

Content of the Methods Section

There is no definitive way to design and conduct focus group research (Morgan, 2010; Barbour, 2007). What is most important is transparency in reporting how the focus group study was conducted and, perhaps more importantly, the rationale for the methodological decisions made. The methods section provides the opportunity to demonstrate that the study was conducted with methodological rigor that supports the validity of the results presented. It is the section of the research report most heavily scrutinized by those assessing the overall quality of the research. Given that the study results arise out of the research methods applied, this is a critical section of any research report. Word limits often restrict the amount of detail that can be provided. Therefore, the methods section needs to be concise and comprehensive.

A typical methods section provides some background on the study setting and research design, details about study participants and their recruitment, a description of the process of data collection and analysis, how ethical issues were managed, and any limitations of the study. It can be useful to begin the methods section with an overview of the research design and methods of data collection to set the context for the details that follow. The structure, length, and style of the methods section varies by the target audience and type of publication (e.g., journal article, research report). Discussed next are suggestions on the content of a methods section with a focus on writing for academic publications. Details of what to include and why are presented, as are common writing pitfalls and challenges; examples of writing particular sections are shown by using extracts from published focus group research.

Study Setting

A methods section needs not only to "set the scene" of the study by describing where the research was conducted (e.g., country, city, region), but also to justify why this setting was the most appropriate for this particular study. Many studies identify the study location but fail to indicate why this location was selected for the study. The description of the study setting typically appears either in the background or methods section of the research document.

Describing characteristics of the study site provides important contextual information, so that the study findings can be understood against the context in which the research was conducted. It is common to briefly outline broad social and demographic features of the study site and then highlight any conditions or characteristics that are particularly relevant to the study topic. For example, a study about family planning behavior may describe women's limited access to contraception at the study site because of policy restrictions (e.g., a woman must be married, abortion services are illegal in the region). Similarly, a study on access to safe water may highlight that safe water sources are not maintained at the study site leading to residents collecting contaminated water from other sources. The extract below shows a concise description of a study site from focus group research on community and religious perspectives on the prevention of type 2 diabetes among the British Bangladeshi population. Therefore, the description highlights the broad socio-cultural context, religious identity, and diabetes prevalance of the study community.

> This study took place in the London borough of Tower Hamlets, one of the most densely populated, multi-ethnic and socio-economically deprived areas in the UK, where the age adjusted prevalence of diabetes is 5.9%. The Bangladeshi population comprised 34% of the borough in 2001, is the largest Sylheti community outside Bangalsesh, with many classifying themselves as Sunni Muslims. Religion has a strong visible presence in the locality although there are dynamic sociocultural trends influencing the link between faith and identity. (Grace, Begum, Subhani, Kopelman, & Greenhalgh, 2008, p. 1)

A longer description of a study site in South Africa is shown below. This study focused on adolescent sexual behavior in rural

South Africa in an area with high HIV prevalence. The description of the study site highlights the context of poverty, illiteracy, and unemployment in the province where the focus group study was conducted, because this impacts the social and sexual behavior of young people, which is the focus of the study itself.

> This study was conducted in Mankweng, about 30 kilometers east of Limpopo Province's capital city, Polokwane. Mankweng settlements consist mostly of periurban townships, tribal villages and informal settlements, where large families live under relatively deprived conditions, lacking a satisfactory water supply and sanitation, and having inadequate access to basic services. A significant percentage of the labor force is unemployed and there are few possibilities for employment. This forces many adults to leave their families in search of employment elsewhere, mainly in the mining industry or the Limpopo farms but also in other sectors available to less educated people. This labor migration has profound implications in terms of reduced social cohesion and many young people have to take on parental responsibilities. The population is very young, with approximately 60% under the age of 18 years. More than a third of those aged 20 years and older in Limpopo Province have not received sufficient education or schooling. Furthermore, educational attainment in the province is below the national level and in Mankweng the illiteracy rate is approximately 10%. As one of the poorest provinces in South Africa, Limpopo spends less than the national average on health services and the HIV prevalence among the poor and disadvantaged population is high, at approximately 19.3%. (Ragnarsson, Onya, Thorson, Ekstrom, & Aaro, 2008, p. 740–741)

It is also useful to indicate how the study site was selected and what informed site selection. Was site selection informed by empirical data, for example study sites were selected because they had the highest concentration of the phenonenon of interest? Was site selection informed by key informants in the region because those sites are where the issues of interest are known to be present? Was the focus group study linked to previous research conducted at the same location? Studies conducted across multiple study sites need additional description to understand differences between each site and reasons for conducting the study in several locations. It is common, for example, to select both rural and urban study sites or sites with or without certain characteristics (e.g., services, facilities, and so forth) to identify how the phenomenon of interest differs in contrasting settings. The extract below provides a detailed justification for the selection of two contrasting school divisions and the selection of individual schools for a focus group study on physical activity.

> Representatives from two local school divisions in a midsized Canadian city worked with the researchers to identify elementary and high schools from two diverse socioeconomic areas of the city. Two high schools that represented the lower socioeconomic areas were selected based on demographic and social characteristics of the neighbourhoods in which the schools were located. These characteristics included community demographics (income levels, unemployment rates), justice information (general crime statistics, young offenders in school, etc), health information (mental health information, alcohol and drug use, etc), and school data (transcience, single parents, absenteeism, etc). We selected the two high schools that represented the higher socioeconomic areas by using data obtained from neighbourhood profiles (e.g., educational attainment, family income, and neighborhood characteristics). Once the four high schools had been selected, two elementary (Grades 1-8) schools located in close proximity to each of the high schools and fulfilling the same low- or high-SES neighbourhood criteria were included in the study. (Humbert et al., 2006, p. 469).

For some studies, the study site may be an institution (e.g., prison, school, hospital); therefore, the nature of the institution is described and why this was specifically selected for the study. Other studies may conduct virtual focus groups by telephone or Internet, whereby there is no specific study site per se to describe. Instead, the focus is on describing the characteristics of the participant group and the logistics of conducting the virtual group discussion. Finally, the date and duration of data collection are typically included. as are details about any collaborating organizations and the their involvement in the study.

Study Design

An important component of the methods section is to identify the overall study design and how focus group discussions fit into the study design selected. Often the study design is not described unless it differs from a typical cross-sectional study design, such as longitudinal research, experimental research design, or mixed methods research design.

Many studies use a typical cross-sectional research design where focus group discussions are the only method of data collection. In this case it is useful to describe why focus group discussions were the most appropriate method of data collection for the study. Other studies may adopt a longitudinal study design that includes multiple episodes of data collection using focus group discussions. For longitudinal research a description of the purpose of each round of focus group discussions is warranted and whether the study is a panel design that uses the same focus group participants each time or uses different participants. It is also common for focus group discussions to be included in mixed methods research designs that combine several qualitative methods (e.g., focus group discussions and in-depth interviews) or use both qualiative and quantitative methods (e.g., focus group discussions and a population survey).

In mixed methods research, it is particularly important to identify how each method of data collection contributes to the research objectives. This may involve highlighting the specific research aim where focus group data will contribute, or explaining how focus group data may inform the design of other components of the study. For example, data from focus group discussions may be used to design elements of a household survey or to identify the questions to include on an in-depth interview guide. Too often studies use mixed methods without a clear description of the purpose of each method or their contribution to the overall research objectives. This is a particular issue when both in-depth interviews and focus group discussions are used in a study with no description of an overall study design to describe why both methods were needed, the different data that each would produce, and how these data contribute to different aspects of the research question. This description is warranted to dispel criticism of data redundancy and to demonstrate relevant application of each method to the overall study purpose.

A common problem is that a study design may be named but it remains unclear why this study design was appropriate for the particular study. This issue can arise in research that uses less common study designs, such as longitudinal, case study, ethnography, or mixed methods research designs. A reader needs sufficient information to help them answer the question: "why is the study design used suitable for this particular study?" Therefore, a brief statement may be included to justify the study design selected in relation to the research objectives.

Study Population and Participant Recruitment

The characteristics of the study population and how they were recruited are critical components of the research methods section. Sufficient detail should be provided for a reader to understand the exact study population and how study participants were recruited from this population. A reader should be able to broadly repeat the process of recruitment with the information provided; however, many research reports provide insufficient detail about these aspects of the research process.

A clear description of the study population is needed. Usually the study population is defined in a brief statement, for example, "Study participants were young women aged 15–25 who had received counselling about anorexia from the clinic in the last 12 months. Those who were currently in treatment for the condition were excluded from the study." This statement succinctly identifies the eligibility criteria for participants and the exclusion criterion. Other studies may list each eligibility criterion with a brief statement on why it was important for the particular study. Some studies may have several distinct target groups, such as health providers and patients, or parents and adolescents. Therefore, a description of each target group is needed. Even though the study population is defined at the outset of the study it may have been refined during data collection or an additional target group added as more is learned about the study topic. Describing this iterative process and how it influenced participant recruitment is useful to reflect the circular nature of qualitative research.

Details on the process of participant recruitment are important, but are often omitted from a description of the research methods. Vaughn, Shay Schumm, and Sinagub (1996) reviewed 150 articles reporting focus group methodology and found that most studies neglected to describe participant selection criteria and recruitment procedures, only reporting the number of study participants. Full details of the participant recruitment are needed. It is insufficient to only state that "purposive sampling" was used, because this is a theoretical approach and not a method of recruitment per se. There are many ways to achieve purposive sampling (i.e., snowball recruitment, venue-based recruitment) and these may be applied in multiple ways and be influenced by the context in which they are applied. Therefore, a description of the actual recruitment process and its rationale is warranted. The goal is to provide sufficient detail on the recruitment process to enable readers to judge whether the process used was appropriate, adequate, and rigorous. Therefore, stating that "participants were recruited through a community leader" or "venue-based recruitment was used" provides no further detail on exactly how recruitment was conducted. Although word limits often lead to much methodological detail being omitted, it is still possible to provide a succinct description of the process of participant recruitment. The two extracts below include descriptions of the process of participant recruitment that describe exactly how recruitment was conducted.

A community-based sample of African American women was recruited in a large metropolitan area in the south eastern region of the United States. Purposive sampling was used to obtain a sample of women who were diverse in age and educational levels. Each scheduled group was designed to be homogenous in age and educational background, to bring individuals together who have shared life experiences... Flyers were distributed strategically at locations including a historically Black university campus, a community college, a women's health clinic, several government agencies (e.g., local health department), hair salons, local libraries, African American women's civic organization meetings, and a local recreation centre and local cultural centre (both of which served the local African American community). Interested persons were instructed on the flyers to contact, via telephone or email, the principal investigator (PI) to learn more about the study. Prospective participants were informed that the study objective was to learn more about how African American women experience and cope with stress; individuals were told that participation would include a 2 hour focus group and brief follow-up contact, and that participants would receive $30 as compensation for

their time. After a telephone-based informed consent process, participants completed a screening questionnaire to
determine eligibility and to obtain demographic information for the purposive sampling. If a woman chose to participate in the study, she was informed that research personnel
would contact her to schedule a date, time, and location.
(Woods-Giscombe, 2010, p. 670)

Recruitment took place at four antiretroviral clinics geo-
graphically dispersed throughout southern Malawi. Three of
the clinics were situated in rural villages, and one was in an
urban setting. Whenever the researchers were present to do
a focus group at a site, the clinic nurses would ask the first
six women who were at least 18 years of age if they would be
interested in participating in a focus group. On every occa-
sion, that is, for three focus groups at each clinic site all the
women approached expressed interest in participating in the
study. Following recruitment, the first author provided each
woman with additional details about the study, including
the limits of confidentiality in focus groups, and obtained
informed consent. None of the women participating with-
drew from the study. For their participation, women received
a modest nonmonetary gift of a packet of sugar, a bar of soap
and a packet of salt. (Mkandawire-Valhmu & Stevens, 2010,
p. 687)

Some studies use several methods of participant recruitment or
different recruitment strategies at different study sites, in particular at urban and rural study sites or for different methods of data
collection used in the study (e.g., in-depth interviews and focus
group discussions). It is not a limitation to use different recruitment strategies in a study; on the contrary, it provides an indication that recruitment strategies are selected as appropriate to the
study context, therefore the description of each recruitment strategy should be included.

It is essential to identify the number of focus groups conducted
in the study. The overall number of focus groups in any study
is likely to be small, often less than 20 groups. Given that this
may seem to be a small sample for readers more familiar with

quantitative research, it is important to deflect the expectation of a representative sample, therefore avoiding the primary objection to qualitative studies that the findings are not generalizable (Belgrave, Zablotsky, & Guadagno, 2002). Indicate that the goal of participant recruitment is inductive discovery of the research issues and not generalizability, and justify why a representative sample is not sought or appropriate. Sample size is a linchpin for scientific research, therefore it is important to indicate how and why the sample size is appropriate for the study. Some studies use theoretical sampling to guide participant recruitment to provide diversity in study participants, and this should be clearly described. The concept of "saturation" determines an adequate sample size in qualitative research, therefore a clear explanation or empirical evidence that saturation (or data redundancy) was achieved is warranted (Guest, MacQueen, & Namey, 2012; Giacomini & Cook, 2000; Bluff, 1997). If saturation did not determine the number of focus groups in the study, a description of how the sample size was determined is needed, for example by using other evidence-based studies as a guide, or indicating budget constraints, logistical considerations, or other reasons. Some aspects of participant recruitment are conducted for pragmatic reasons and these too need to be included. Therefore, describing conceptual and pragmatic influences on the sample size provides transparency in the logic, decisions, and practical constraints on the study.

Given that homogeneity in participant characteristics is important in individual focus group discussions, state exactly how this was achieved and by which criteria participants were homogeneous and how they were heterogeneous. If diversity was built into the study design at the outset by segmenting focus groups by certain characteristics (e.g., age, gender, location), state this clearly and indicate the number of groups conducted per strata and the rationale for the segmentation used. This information may be presented in narrative or table format. Table 3.1 presents segmentation of the study population in table format for a mixed methods study using focus group discussions and in-depth interviews that were segmented by gender (male, female); location (urban, rural); and length of membership in a microcredit group (new, short-term, long-term). The table highlights the number

Table 3.1

Segmentation of Focus Group Discussions and In-Depth Interviews

	New Members (<6 months)	Short-Term Members (1–2 years)	Established Members (5+ years)	Total No. Group Discussions and Interviews
Focus Group Discussions				
Urban site (women)	1	1	1	3 groups
Urban site (men)	1	—	1	2 groups
Rural site (women)	1	1	1	3 groups
Rural site (men)	1	—	1	2 groups
In-Depth Interviews				
Urban site (women)	3	3	3	9 interviews
Rural site (women)	3	3	3	9 interviews

Note: The number in each cell represents the number of interviews or group discussions.

Source: Reproduced with permission from M. Hennink and D. McFarland, "A Delicate Web: Household Changes in Health Behaviour Enabled by Microcredit in Burkina Faso," 2013, *Global Public Health*, *8*(2), 144–158.

of focus group discussions conducted by each stratum, and the reasons for segmentation by these criteria were described in the narrative.

The extract below provides an effective narrative justification for the segmentation of focus groups among the study population of African Americans with renal disease.

We conducted focus group meetings involving African American and non-African American patients with end stage renal disease and their family members or friends for the purpose of eliciting their experiences with decision-making concerning their choice of RRT [Renal Replacement Therapy]. We hypothesized that participants' perspective on decision making about RRT initiation might differ according to their ethnicity/race, as well as their status as a patient or family member. We also hypothesized that experiences with RRT initiation might vary according to treatment modality (hemodialysis, peritoneal dialysis, transplant). We therefore conducted focus groups stratified by race/ethnicity, patient / family member status and current treatment modality. (Sheu et al., 2012, p. 998)

Data Collection

The process of data collection needs to be described in detail. This is important because of the flexible nature of qualitative research whereby data collection may evolve iteratively as the study progresses. Belgrave and colleagues (2002, p. 1430–1431) describe this process and how it may appear to readers; "as we begin to make sense of the phenomenon under investigation, we might change our approach, change our focus, add research sites, even develop new strategies or tools...However, this strength can appear as a weakness. We can leave [readers] with the impression that we...flew by seat of our pants, with little idea of our destination." They go on to say that these impressions are avoidable by providing a transparent description of the data collection process and its rationale. If data collection proceeded in an iterative way this needs to be described at the outset, in particular how data collection was empirically guided and which aspects of data collection followed the iterative process.

All methods of data collection used in the study need to be stated and a rationale given for each method used. One indicator of research quality is the selection of <u>appropriate</u> methods of data collection for the research objectives; therefore, state why focus group discussions were suitable for the specific objectives of the study. If multiple methods were used, the purpose of each method should be stated. For example, a study on stigma related to obesity may use focus group discussions to identify community perceptions of obese people, and use in-depth interviews with obese people to identify individual experiences of stigma. Each research method therefore has a clear and distinct purpose related to the overall research objective. The example below provides a clear and concise justification for the selection of focus group discussions in a study on HIV vaccine acceptability in South Africa.

We selected an exploratory qualitative study design to allow us the opportunity to approach the topic broadly, given that there is little existing knowledge on this topic. We chose to explore post-trial HIV vaccine acceptability through FGDs because this method allows for expression of views and for opinions about products within the broader social context from which the participants come. This group experience replicates the experience study participants might have in decision making around this topic outside of the research setting, and is therefore more useful than the collection of individual perceptions might be. (MacPhail, Sayles, Cummingham, & Newman, 2012, p. 669–670)

It is also important to indicate who collected the data, whether this was the authors or members of a field team. A brief description of the characteristics of the focus group moderator and note-taker is typically included, because a moderator can influence the focus group dynamic and the data generated (discussed in next section on Reflexivity). A typical description may include how many moderators were used, whether they were gender matched to the focus group participants, and whether they shared the same cultural background. It is also useful to indicate whether moderators were experienced in focus group research or were trained specifically for the study. Other relevant details may include the language skills of moderators where focus group discussions were conducted in another language. For example,

The group interview... was moderated by one of the authors (a 29-year-old White female graduate student with previous interview experience). (Jette, Wilson, & Sparks, 2007, p. 327)

The research team for phase one of the study was composed of a female nurse researcher who had basic competence in Spanish and was experienced in conducting focus groups, a bilingual translator from the United States, and two local bilingual research assistants with previous experience working as health clinic assistants. The principal investigator served as the focus group facilitator. (Cooper & Yarbrough, 2010, p. 647)

A description of the discussion guide used to collect data is a key component of the methods section. Indicate how the guide was developed, for example questions may have been developed from concepts in the literature, previous empirical research, or in collaboration with colleagues familiar with the study context or community. A list of topics covered on the discussion guide is usually provided, so that readers can understand what was asked in the group discussion and whether certain questioning strategies were used to improve data validity (e.g., recall strategies for retrospective questions). Some studies include the wording of select questions asked, where these form a critical part of the analysis and research goals. If activities were part of the focus group, these should also be described and the type of data generated by the activity. It is usual to indicate how the research instrument was piloted and any resulting changes made to the instrument. The research instrument may be included in the appendix of a research report, but is rarely included in a journal article. Below are two extracts that show how the description of the research instrument was reported. The first example highlights the theoretical framework that influenced the questioning strategy (the ecologic model) and the second example describes how questions were posed in the group discussion to acknowledge they were being asked in a group setting and to protect individual confidentiality.

> The focus group interviews were centered on one open ended question: 'If you could be the one in charge of increasing the physical activity level of kids your age, what would you do?' We used a number of questions designed around the three components of the ecological model to prompt the open ended question. Examples of such questions included 'Would you need to be skilled to participate in this activity or program?' (intrapersonal); 'Would you do this activity alone or with friends?' (social); and 'Where would this activity be done?' (environmental)... (Humbert et al., 2006, p. 470)

> Data were collected using a semi structured topic guide that addressed the key issues around vaccine acceptability. After some discussion of vaccines in general, we asked participants relating specifically to HIV vaccines: What have you heard about vaccines for HIV/AIDS? What are the reasons that you or your close friends would want to be vaccinated against HIV/AIDS? What are the reasons that you or your close friends would not want to be vaccinated against

HIV/AIDS? How would being vaccinated change you or your close friends' sexual behavior? Participants were asked to discuss their own views and their perceptions of the views of others in their communities to get a range of responses but also to protect the confidentiality of those not wishing to disclose their own potential behaviors. (MacPhail et al., 2012, p. 670)

Including logistical details about data collection also provides useful context about how the focus groups were conducted. Indicate where focus groups were held, whether they were conducted in community locations, how privacy was maintained, how seating was arranged, and any drawbacks of the location used. Indicate the length of the group discussion and explain any particularly long (more than 2 hours) or short (less than an hour) groups. If the group was conducted in another language this needs to be stated. Include whether participants were provided with refreshments, incentives, or a payment to attend. Any difficulties encountered in conducting the group discussions need to be highlighted and whether these were mitigated, because they may influence the quality of the data generated. A description of how the group discussions were recorded is essential. Typically focus group discussions are recorded using an audio-recording device (e.g., digital or tape recorder) or by a note-taker. If a recording device was not used, indicate the reasons why and state how data were then generated.

Reflexivity

Qualitative research involves intense interaction with study participants and uses flexible research instruments, which can lead to a greater potential for the researcher to influence data collected, compared with a fixed-format quantitative survey. Furthermore, the researcher's background, position, or presentation can also influence data collection and interpretation (Green & Thorogood, 2009; Berg, 2007; Hesse-Biber & Leavy, 2006; Finlay & Gough, 2003; Pillow, 2003). Qualitative researchers are therefore advised to describe the characteristics of those involved in data collection and analysis and highlight any potential effect this may have had on data generated, this is known as *reflexivity*. Reflexivity therefore needs to be considered in writing qualitative research to make explicit any potential influences of the researchers or the research process on data produced. Reporting reflexivity is also important to demonstrate an understanding of the interpretive paradigm, the influence of subjectivity, and how it was managed throughout the research process, thereby contributing to the rigor of the study. Reflexivity is typically reported in the methods section, and the level of detail is influenced by the broad paradigm underlying the research discipline or academic journal, whereby social sciences typically require more detail on this than biomedical science (Corbin & Strauss, 2008; Finlay & Gough, 2003; Lynch, 2000).

Two aspects of refexivity, highlighted by Hesse-Biber and Leavy (2006), are commonly reported: personal and interpersonal reflexivity. *Personal reflexivity* involves reflecting on the researchers' own background and assumptions and how these influenced the research process and data generated. For example, the socio-cultural background, gender, training, or presentation of a focus group moderator sends certain unconscious signals to participants about this person, whereas the researcher's own beliefs and assumptions about the study population influences their questioning strategies and interpretation of the group discussion. Therefore, a methods section typically highlights the background characteristics of those involved in data collection and analysis and highlights any clear (or potential) influences on the data collected and whether (and how) these were managed.

The extracts from focus group studies below show how researchers acknowledged personal reflexivity by describing the potential influence of the moderator's characteristics on participants, and whether this was managed in any way.

It is particularly important to point out for this report that although the first author is a Malawian woman and has experienced understanding of the social and cultural context of the women's lives, her educational background and social class required her to make efforts to flatten the hierarchical power inherent in the process of research... For instance, she dressed in clothing common in the context, limited use of technologies with which the women were unfamiliar, prioritized verbal over written communication and used the inclusive first-person plural *we* in posing questions. (Mkandawire-Valhmu & Stevens, 2010, p. 686)

Recognizing that the role of the facilitator in the data collection, we selected a young African woman fluent in all three languages to moderate the discussions in the belief that her age, gender and race would counter the educational distance between herself and the discussion participants. This focus on reflexivity has been noted as vital in other qualitative data collection using FGDs. (MacPhail et al., 2012, p. 670)

Although I was no longer employed by the correctional system, my social location as a White, middle-class woman with formal education allied me with the authority of the institution [a US prison]. It is likely that my status as White and middle class and the prison environment both influenced and shaped the participants' narratives. (Pollack, 2003, p. 466)

Interpersonal reflexivity involves reviewing the setting of the group discussions and the interpersonal dynamic within the group and between the moderator and participants, which may have influenced data produced. For example, power dynamics may have emerged in a group discussion, interruptions to the group may have influenced participation, or there may have been issues with the location where the groups were held or with the level of rapport development achieved. These issues may influence data generated and are important to note in the description of research methods. The first two examples below are from a focus group study among prison inmates and staff and demonstrate reporting of interpersonal reflexivity. The first quotation indicates how the situational influence of the prison context may have influenced participants' contributions, whereas the second describes how potential power dynamics between the researchers and participants were diverted. The third example shows how reflexivity on group dynamics was reported in a study among participants with serious mental health issues, who were recruited to share their experiences on receiving support services.

During one group interview, for example, the primary investigator took a visible step to ensure that members of the inmate peer staff refrained from walking into the area where the interviews were being conducted as their presence was inhibiting. This small gesture was interpreted by the inmates that the primary researcher was independent, understood the inmate or convict code of conduct and its influences on the tenets of daily prison life, and was willing to protect them during the data-gathering phase; this resulted in a noticeable increase in the depth of discussion and the number of inmates participating. (Patenaude, 2004, p. 78S)

On numerous occasions during each group interview, it was necessary to reassure the participants that the research team was independent of ADC [Arkansas Department of Correction] and was seeking ways to improve the substance abuse treatment program. (Patenaude, 2004, p. 78S).

In all focus groups the women mainly directed comments to me [moderator] and were often reluctant to discuss issues amongst themselves. This was possibly a reflection of the women's poor communication and social skills, and their lack of experience of sharing ideas in a group... Whilst this dynamic became increasingly evident as the study progressed, it was difficult to see how it could be resolved... Whilst the level of verbal interaction in the focus groups was low, there was evidence of other types of interaction amongst the women. In particular, there appeared to be considerable empathy between the women, nonverbal acknowledgement of shared experiences, and they were frequently very supportive towards one another. (Owen, 2001, p. 655–656)

A common concern about reporting reflexivity is how far to go. What is important is to find a balance between demonstrating reflexivity and becoming overly analytical on potential influences on the study. Finlay (2002, p. 541) states that "we need to strike a balance, striving for enhanced self-awareness but eschewing navel gazing." Similarly, Guest et al. (2012, p. 252) fairly argue that "the researcher, research process and research context can affect *all* types of data collection... it doesn't seem productive or fair to ask practitioners of qualitative reserch to discuss reflexivity or response bias to a greater degree than researchers in other disciplines. In line with good overall scientific practice we therefore recommend that qualitative researchers simply report the known potential for, and measures taken to minimise, relevant biases in their studies, as one would with any scientific study." Researchers values and self-identity may also be ingrained within individuals, therefore some level of reflexivity in writing research findings is important to bring forth a greater sense of self-awareness on the researcher's role in shaping data generation. Reflexivity is needed in all research studies to legitimize, to validate, and to question the research process (Pillow, 2003).

Data Analysis

The description of data analysis continues to be one of the weakest areas of published qualitative research (Guest et al., 2012). Several issues are common weaknesses in reporting data analysis. First, data analysis is often treated as a "black box" whereby analytic procedures are simply absent from written reports. In other situations only a broad analytic approach is mentioned with no detail on the analytic tasks, procedures, or decisions made to support the findings presented. For example, stating only that "thematic analysis was used" provides insuffiecent information about how data were actually analyzed and the procedural steps taken to ensure validity of the study findings. Unfortunately, articles with these critical omissions are still published. Second, at times analytic methods are reported incorrectly. As qualitative research increases in popularity specific analytic terminology has become familiar and appears in research reports without evidence that the task or approach stated was actually used. This is perhaps seen most often in studies claiming to use the "grounded theory" approach, yet the analytic tasks described or the nature of the results presented do not follow grounded theory and most fall short of theory development. Third, some research reports present a "textbook" description of analytic processes resulting in a generic outline of procedural steps in analysis, with no indication of how analytic tasks were applied to the specific study data. These limitations on reporting data analysis have critical omissions that make it difficult to judge the quality of the analysis and validity of the results. Therefore, including procedural detail that is specific to the study data is a critical component in reporting data analysis. Reporting of data analysis also differs by the analytic approach used. Below are some general guidelines on what may be reported in a comprehensive description of data analysis in focus group research.

For readers unfamiliar with qualitative research, the analytic procedures used need to be made explicit and clear so that readers can follow the analytic process and thinking that led to the conclusions presented. Belgrave et al. (2002) make this point succintly: "if our strategies for selecting research participants and collecting data are somewhat unfamiliar to quantitative [readers], our means of analyzing data verge on the incomprehensible... to tell a quantitative [reader] that 'categories will emerge from the data' or that you 'will develop themes' is to tell him or her virtually nothing" (p. 1435–1436). The description of data analysis therefore needs to be sufficiently transparent to be understood by almost any scientific audience. Rather than relying on certain terminology to be self-evident of an analytic task (e.g., codes, categories, constant comparison), explain what was actually done in clear and simple words to enable the analytic process to become meaningful to those unfamiliar with this approach. Some suggestions on areas of greater transparency are described next.

Describe how data were prepared for analysis

Indicate whether written transcripts were developed from the group discussions, if these transcripts were verbatim or in another format, and how data were cleaned and checked for accuracy. State whether field notes or additonal data from the group discussions were part of the analysis and the form of these additional data. (e.g., drawings, pile sorts, and so forth). If transcription also involved translation of the discussion, describe how the translation was conducted and verified. If a written transcript was not developed, provide the reasons. State the name and version of any computer package that was used for textual data analysis and describe exactly how it was used in analysis. Even when software is used it is still necessary to document the analytic steps undertaken, because software for qualitative data does not actually do the analysis itself, rather it provides tools that allow researchers to manipulate the textual data in various ways to facilitate analysis.

Identify the overall analytic approach used and the rationale for selecting it

Grounded theory, thematic analysis, conversation analysis, and content analysis are examples of distinct approaches to textual data analysis, each with a different analytic focus and distinct analytic tasks. Providing a rationale for selecting the analytic approach used provides evidence of research quality, which begins with selecting an analytic approach appropriate for the research objectives. It is not sufficient to only identify the analytic approach used without providing the procedural detail on exactly how analysis was then conducted. Analytic processes vary and there exist adaptations of several approaches, therefore procedural details of the analytic tasks conducted are important. A comprehensive description of data analysis provides an audit trail of all analytic tasks conducted, begining with data preparation and each subsequent analytic task conducted. This demonstrates analytic rigor and how the study findings presented were derived. The analytic description also needs to be complete. For example, some studies using thematic analysis or grounded theory only provide details about data preparation (e.g., developing codes and coding data) but then fail to describe how the coded data were then analyzed, because coding is only one task in the anaytic process of these approaches. Therefore, a comprehensive description of all analytic steps and procedures is needed.

Describe how analytic tasks were applied to the study data
Avoid presenting a generic description of data analysis by describing how analytic tasks were applied to the particular study. For example, indicate whether certain concepts from the literature were used as codes, identify which intercoder assessment procedures were used and their outcome, describe specific comparisons made across data, provide examples of inductive categories developed, or detail the components of a conceptual framework developed. These details provide specificity on how analytic tasks were applied to the study data. In addition, a description of analytic reasoning makes transparent how certain concepts were developed from the data or why links between certain issues are important. Overall, what is needed is a transparent description of the analytic tasks used and the analytic reasoning to provide a comprehensive description of data anlysis.

Describe how study findings were validated
Describing measures to ensure the validity of the study findings is often overlooked in the research methods section. Indicate any techniques used to ensure that the issues identified, concepts developed, or explanations presented are empirically grounded in the study data. These details are critical to demonstrate that the results presented are valid and based on systematic data analysis involving effective validity checks, and not subjective interpretation. This information may comprise a separate paragraph or validity checks may be interspersed with the description of the

methodological tasks. Strategies for qualitative data validity and reliability are described in Chapter 5.

Ethical Issues

It is usual to indicate ethical approval of the study and how ethical issues were adressed throughout the research process. Issues of consent and permission need to be described in the research methods. For example, state how informed consent was received from participants (e.g., oral or written), and how permission to record the group discussion was sought. In addition, describe how participants were informed that their involvement in the focus group is voluntary and they have a right to leave the discussion at any time. Confidentiality and anonymity can be particular concerns in focus group research because of the group nature of data collection. Therefore, indicate measures taken to maintain confidentiality of the information shared in the group, and how data records were secured. State how participant identities were protected. Also describe how anonymity of participants was managed in reporting the study findings. Indicate whether participants received any incentive or payment for participation in the group discussion and how potential coersion was curbed. Additional ethical issues may relate to the discussion of sensitive topics, such as how potential harm to participants was minimized (e.g., in question phrasing, provision of support materials).

Study Limitations

It is routine to indicate any limitations of the study that influence how the study findings are read and understood. The main focus here is on the methodological limitations of the study, such as limitations of the study design, selection of participants, data collection issues, and so on. However, a common pitfall is that generic drawbacks of qualitative research are reported rather than the limitations of the particular study. Simply stating the drawbacks of the qualitative approach (e.g., small sample size) or limitations of focus group research (e.g., reduced confidentiality) is not informative because these are generally well known and are anticipated at the outset of the study. It is more appropriate to report limitations of the study per se, such as a study that was only conducted with women, thereby the exclusion of male perspectives was a limitation, or a study conducted only in rural areas is limited by the exclusion of data from urban participants. Specific omission may also be described, such as certain topics not discussed in the focus groups that may in hindsight have yielded fruitful data. Other limitations may include unforeseen logistical issues that arose during data collection and curtailed the original study design, or compromised the quality of data collected. Describing these limitations allows readers to understand the boundaries of the study when reading the study findings. It is also good practice to indicate whether (and how) study limitations were minimized. Although some methodological limitations simply need to be stated, other issues may have arisen during data collection and were mitigated in some way.

The extracts below report the limitations section of two separate focus group studies. Each extract reports limitations specific to the study design (not generic limitations of qualitative research). For example, each describes the potential limitations in how researchers structured the composition of focus groups (e.g., limitations of using groups of participants with mixed language skills in the first example and using single-gender group composition in the second). Each example also indicates how potential limitations were minimized. The first example also indicates the parameters in which the study findings can be relevant to other settings to deflect the limitation that qualitative findings lack generalizability.

> Several considerations must be kept in mind when interpreting the findings derived from this study. First, we offer a caveat related to language. Although the inclusion of multiple ethnic-linguistic groupings enabled us to hear about the experience of service users who are not often included in other studies, important themes or cultural references may have been 'lost in translation.' In a broader sense, we also noted the possibility of 'linguistic disparities' across focus groups, with members of some groups expressing their experiences more eloquently than members of other groups. Second, we acknowledge that we seek transferability rather than generalizability... Accordingly, the findings are applicable to contexts that are similar to the one in which this study was undertaken, that is, urban environments in which individuals with mental health problems of diverse cultures use formal treatment programs or peer support groups. Third, we recognise that the findings reflect the subjective experiences of the study participants and the cultural communities

about which they spoke. (Wong, Sands, & Solomon, 2010, p. 658–659)

We acknowledge that there are limitations to the data used in this article. We collected data in this study through focus group discussions, which might have allowed for overrepresentation of some research participants who might have dominated the conversation and influenced the overall dynamics of the groups. We made attempts to account for this through ensuring that all comments in the transcripts were accountable to individuals for tracking, and by using a facilitator skilled in managing group dynamics. The information might also be influenced by the decision to use single-gender FGDs, although we did this to increase participant comfort with a potentially difficult and sensitive topic. We did not use a formal translation and back translation process for the topic guide, given that FGDs should be reflexive and not dependent on formally structured questions. This might have resulted in errors in interpretation that we did not identify, although attempts were made to limit this through in-depth discussion of the FGD topic guide with the facilitator, specifically examining the language to be used. (MacPhail et al., 2012, p. 675)

Readers may also expect some indication on the extent to which study findings can be transferred to other settings or similar population groups. In general, population level generalizability is not within the scope of focus group research; however, transferability of the findings from qualitative research is typically achieved in the "conceptual transferability of the concepts generated, rather than the statistical representativeness of the sample" (Green & Thorogood, 2009, p. 267). Therefore, it is useful to highlight any concepts generated from the study that may have wider applicability and to indicate their potential transferability.

Finally, if all the advice in this chapter were heeded in writing the methods section of a qualitative study, the document would go well beyond any prescribed word limits. Therefore, careful discretion is needed in deciding where greater detail or justification is required for a particular study. This is primarily guided by the target audience and the purpose of the research itself. However, perhaps the core advice of this chapter is the following: first, to adhere to the interpretive paradigm when writing qualitative research methods, even though the procedures may need to be explained; and second, to become practiced at concisely conveying scientific procedures while maintaining analytic depth.

Key Points

....

* There is no single way to conduct focus group research; therefore, it is necessary to provide transparency on the research process and methodological decisions that shaped the study outcomes.

* The methods section is a critical component of the research report and needs to simultaneously describe the research process, set the context of the study, and reflect the quality of the study.

* The research methods section needs to not only state *what* was done, but also *how* it was done and *why* it was done this way.

* Writing the research methods needs to reflect the interpretive paradigm within which focus research is conducted, in terms of describing the research process, applying methodological concepts, and using appropriate terminology.

* A challenge in writing the methods section is to write concisely yet provide the necessary procedural detail and methodological justifications that give the study scientific credibility.

* The methods section may include a description of various contexts, such as the theoretical context of the research problem, the socio-cultural context of the study, and the methodological context of data collection.

* The research methods section is inevitably shaped by the target audience and their requirements.

* The research methods section typically includes a description of the study setting, research design, participant recruitment, data collection and analysis, ethical issues, and study limitations.

4

WRITING FOCUS GROUP RESULTS

WRITING THE RESULTS of qualitative research is a very different experience from writing quantitative research findings. In part, this is because of the nature of the data being reported (textual not numerical data) and also the different role that writing plays in qualitative research. Writing the results of qualitative research is much more than simply presenting the outcomes of data analysis; it is a component of analysis itself.

Writing the study findings also leads to the final outcome of the research. This aspect of writing is the focus of this chapter. In writing the study findings consider the key messages of the study, the intended audience, and the most effective way to present the study findings. This requires presentation strategies that reflect the nature of the qualitative evidence and also effectively interpret this research evidence. Effectively presenting textual data and demonstrating valid interpretations of the data can be challenging. It can also be difficult to present qualitative research findings in a concise, coherent, and compelling way and still maintain the character and complexity of the data. As with Chapter 3, the focus of this chapter is on writing results for academic audiences; however, the guidance can also be applied to writing for other audiences.

This chapter begins with a description of some of the challenges in writing qualitative study results, highlighting particular issues in reporting focus group data. This is followed by guidance on different aspects to consider when writing focus group results. These include the importance of structure and presenting a coherent argument, the use of quotations, and how to present interaction found in focus group data. Visual presentation strategies are described and how to reflect context throughout the study findings. A key aspect of writing focus group results is demonstrating that the issues reported are "grounded," or well evidenced by data, and strategies for grounding the findings are described. Finally, focus group study findings are often presented as part of mixed methods research; therefore, guidance for the presentation of mixed methods study results is provided. Several common pitfalls in writing focus group results are highlighted throughout the chapter with suggestions to overcome these pitfalls.

Challenges in Writing Focus Group Results

The overall purpose of the results section is to present the study findings in a clear and compelling way in response to the research objectives. In this way writing the results of qualitative research is similar to reporting quantitative research. However, qualitative research and focus group discussions in particular generate a different type of evidence to quantitative studies, which present different writing challenges. Writing the results of focus group research shares many of the challenges of writing qualitative results in general, yet the group nature of data collection provides additional opportunities for presentation of results. Reporting focus group data also needs to respect the tradition in which data were collected and capitalize on the strengths of this approach. Focus group data offer the opportunity to identify variation, explain nuances, and present a group narrative, all of which can be exploited in writing the results. Writing study results can seem challenging at first, but can also become one of the most rewarding aspects of the research process. Some of the challenges in reporting focus group results are highlighted next and reflected throughout this chapter.

Writing as Data Analysis

One of the initial challenges in writing focus group results stems from understanding the circular process of writing as a component of data analysis. In qualitative research writing the study results is an integral part of data analysis and not simply a final task of "writing up" the study findings. Wolcott (2001, p. 22) states that in qualitative research "writing is thinking... [or] one form that thinking can take." Writing the results of qualitative research is actually a circular process whereby one begins to identify the study findings and the core messages from the study, which inevitably generates further questions about the data, identifies clarifications needed, or gaps in the emerging study findings, and this leads back to the data for further analysis to refine the study findings. This process may be repeated multiple times creating a circular process between writing, further analysis, and back to writing, each time gaining a clearer understanding of the research issues and how to effectively report these. In this way, "the act of writing is a rich and analytic process as you find yourself not only attempting to explain and justify your ideas but also developing them" (Rapley, 2011, p. 286). Coffey and Atkinson (1996, p. 109, cited in Ritchie & Lewis, 2003, p. 288) describe this circular process; they state that "writing and representing is a vital way of thinking about one's data. Writing makes us think about data in new and different ways. Thinking about how to represent our data forces us to think about the meanings and understandings, voices and experiences present in the data. As such writing actually deepens our level of analytic endeavor. Analytical ideas are developed and tried out in the process of writing and representing." Therefore, writing the study results is another analytic tool to further interpret, refine, and conceptualize data, and is thus conducted simultaneously with further exploration of data. This circular process can seem confusing for those more familiar with the linear approach of research whereby data analysis and writing the results are seen as separate consecutive tasks. Understanding the integration of writing and data analysis is an important first step to writing the results of focus group research. Of course, writing also produces the final product of the research, and is an outcome of this circular process.

Data Reduction

Focus group discussions produce a large volume of data and data reduction is a core challenge in writing the study findings. It can seem overwhelming to write the study results at first because of the large volume of data to synthesize and the difficulty in identifying core findings from the complex range of issues discussed. However, data reduction is an essential precursor to writing the study findings and is achieved initially through data analysis. For example, data analysis identifies core themes or categories of issues in the data, conceptualizes data, or develops a framework for structuring the results, all of which contribute to data reduction. Not all study findings are included in the final report, therefore further data reduction involves identifying the most salient and meaningful study results that respond directly to the research objectives. Data reduction therefore begins to make sense of the research findings and forms the "story" of the data, which helps to effectively structure the study findings. Writing the study results without sufficient data reduction can be extremely challenging. When writing results seems difficult, it is often due to insufficient data analysis to clarify the core issues because they are still obscured within the volume of data. In these situations it is necessary to return to data analysis to gain greater clarity on the study results. Although data reduction is needed before writing the study results, the process of writing can also help to find logic and structure in the study results or identify gaps where further analysis is needed to clarify specific findings (as described previously). Therefore, data analysis leads to data reduction, which facilitates writing the study results.

The results section of a focus group study can be lengthy because results are presented in narrative form (versus a concise table of statistics) and illustrated with quotations, both of which add to the word length of the results. In addition, there is often more interpretive text presented in the results section to help the reader navigate the context and complexities in the issues presented. It can be challenging to synthesize the study findings concisely yet still reflect the depth, variation, and complexity of the issues. The challenge is to reflect the depth and complexity of focus group results, yet manage the word limits prescribed by academic journals. Qualitative research can attract criticism for the presentation of superficial results, when in reality space limits may have constrained presenting issues in fuller detail.

Reporting Group Data

Focus group data are unique in that they can be reported as individual comments from participants or as a collective group narrative, or as interaction data. The challenge is to identify the appropriate way to report the study findings, and whether using different types of reporting may be effective. Most focus group data are treated as individual comments and reported in much the same way as in-depth interview data. This involves presenting comments from individual participants, often grouped under specific topics. This approach is often sufficient to meet the objectives of most research projects. However, focus group data have an added benefit of presenting a group narrative, which reflects the group nature of data collection and its influence on shaping individual comments. Although individual comments may still be reported they are used to provide evidence of a broader collective narrative developed through the group discussion. Focus group data also contain interactive discussion between participants, which provides a unique opportunity to analyze and present interaction data (see Chapter 2 on data analysis). A key challenge is deciding whether (and how) to report interaction between participants. Group interaction itself can become the focus of data analysis whereby the nature of the interaction becomes the analysis. However, group interaction can also be reflected when reporting the issues discussed in the focus group, by presenting extracts of group dialogue around a specific issue. Reporting group interaction adds depth to the issues described, reflects the group environment in which data were generated, and demonstrates how issues are discussed between participants. Reporting issues and the interactive exchange that produced them is a unique and effective way to present focus group research findings. It can also be effective to use an extract of group dialogue to demonstrate the development of a group narrative. A combination of reporting approaches may be used throughout the research report. Effective reporting of focus group results may use various reporting strategies as appropriate to the study findings and the purpose of the study.

Structure and Argument

Another challenge in writing focus group results is to identify a clear structure, argument, or central message to frame the study results. A well-written results section comprises more than a collection of findings but also presents a coherent argument, narrative, or explanation of issues that is based on the study findings.

The underlying structure or argument helps the reader to navigate the findings presented and understand the conclusions stated. A common pitfall in writing focus group research is the absence of a strong structure, argument, or theoretical framework in presenting the study findings. A related concern is that the results section swamps the reader with data, such as presenting multiple or lengthy quotations, with little narrative text to put the data extracts in context or indicate how they contribute to the overall research findings. This equates to presenting the reader with sections of data and letting them make their own conclusions from the evidence presented. Therefore, an effective results section presents a clear structure or argument and uses data judiciously to support a central narrative. Presenting the study results within a clear structure or theoretical framework also reflects comprehensive data analysis and thoughtful conceptualization of the results, which in turn reflects quality research.

There is no set formula for writing qualitative research findings, so the structure of the results section may look very different across various projects. The presentation of qualitative research findings may also differ from a commonly structured academic report. Typically, an academic report begins with a theoretical or conceptual framework, which is used to guide the description of the study design and provides an anchor for the presentation of the study findings. Although this structure is also used in much qualitative research, additionally a qualitative study may have developed a conceptual framework for understanding the study findings. Therefore, rather than beginning with a *theoretical* framework the results section may present an *empirical* framework. Because this is an outcome of the research, it is presented in the results section and may provide the structure for reporting the study results. This structure is contrary to the expected structure for academic writing, and may therefore need a descriptive justification, although it is entirely appropriate for reporting qualitative research.

Presenting Variation

When writing focus group results it is necessary to demonstrate both centrality and diversity in the issues reported, which can be challenging at first. Within the large volume of data that focus group's generate it is common to focus on reporting common issues and typical perspectives, or to report normative behavior. This is warranted and in itself can be a challenge in a large and complex textual data set. However, focus group data are unique in that they collect data with implicit variation because of using a group of participants contributing to a discussion. Although it is not given that this necessarily produces different views, it is likely to uncover some variation, because even when participants broadly agree on an issue they may have different individual experiences or reasoning for that agreement. The absence of any variation is also an important finding to report. Therefore, focus group data provide an opportunity to capture variation and present nuances in the study results in addition to highlighting a dominant or common perspective. Data analysis may go further to explicitly examine certain deviant perspectives, which may be indicative of underlying social issues, and therefore add considerable depth to the study findings. The challenge is not to become restricted by presenting only centrality in the study findings, because unique and important findings can also be found in diversity where focus group data provide some advantage.

Distinguishing Results and Interpretation

A particular challenge in writing focus group study findings is to distinguish between the presentation of results and their interpretation by researchers. Most stages of qualitative research involve simultaneous analysis and interpretation, which can spur deeper reflection on study findings. Although this is a strength of qualitative research, some academic journals, particularly those in the health sciences, often require a separation between the presentation of results and their interpretation. This is imposed in the required structure of articles submitted, which involve writing a results section that focuses on objective reporting of the study findings followed by a discussion section where these findings are interpreted. However, in qualitative research separating the presentation of results from their interpretation may be an artificial divide, because reading qualitative results often requires understanding the context and nuances that shape these study findings. Without an interpretive narrative in the results section qualitative research results may make less sense. Therefore, presenting qualitative research in an objective format that divides reporting of results from their interpretation can present some writing challenges. Academic journals differ in their flexibility to accommodate these aspects of writing qualitative research, so qualitative researchers may need to adapt to writing in this format or indicate in the results section when interpretations (versus results) are being presented. This requires a different style of writing study findings to accommodate the presentation of results as required by academic journals.

Grounding Study Findings

In writing focus group results, it is important to demonstrate that findings are valid and well-grounded in the data. All study findings should be empirically supported through using rigorous analytic techniques, conducting validity checks, and managing interpretive subjectivity. In qualitative research it can be challenging to demonstrate that the results presented are empirically grounded and not the outcome of a researcher's subjective influence. Many reviewers of qualitative studies equate the presentation of quotations as the only evidence that an issue was indeed present in the study data, and therefore question the validity of results where no data extracts are presented. The challenge lies in demonstrating rigor and validity independent of presenting quotations, because this deflects potential criticism that results are unsupported and not empirically grounded in the data. Furthermore, reporting the strategies used to validate the study findings can also provide evidence that the results of focus group research are well supported by empirical data (see Chapter 5 for discussion on demonstrating validity).

Coherence between Results and Methods

The study results should be a logical outcome of the analytic approach applied as stated in the methods section. Coherence between the methods used and results presented is critical and provides an indicator of scientific rigor in the research report. Therefore, clear coherence is needed between what was said in the methods and what was actually done, as presented in the results. For example, if the research methods indicate that the study used a grounded theory approach, then the results section needs to present the concepts developed, theory extended, or conceptual framework that was derived from this approach to textual data analysis. Unfortunately, too many studies apply a methodological label by stating that a particular approach was used when the study results do not reflect the outcome of the stated approach. Grounded theory, narrative analysis, conversational analysis, content analysis, and case study analysis all have a distinct analytic approach that generates a different type of research result. The challenge is to ensure coherence between the methodological approach stated and analytic outcomes presented in the results.

Ethical Reporting of Data

Ethical reporting of focus group study findings can be more challenging than for other types of research, particularly because participant's own words are reported in quotations. Presenting verbatim quotations is a powerful way to directly present the perspectives of study participants. It is a long-standing tradition of focus group research, and reflects the rich contextual detail that makes the study findings unique. However, care is needed to report quotations ethically by not revealing the identity of study participants that could cause potential harm. Although most researchers understand that participant's names should not be reported, there may be other information in a quotation that could inadvertently reveal the identity of participants. This is particularly problematic when presenting research findings in a case study where more fine grain detail or atypical examples are presented compared with comments from individuals in the group discussion, which can be more easily made anonymous. Furthermore, there is an ethical responsibility to represent participant's viewpoints fairly and respectfully, providing a balanced report of the issues discussed without giving undue importance to quotations or viewpoints that may represent atypical positions. Therefore, ethical reporting of focus group data is both critical and challenging.

Writing the Results Section

Beginning to Write Results

Beginning to write the results of focus group research can seem like a daunting task. Focus group data are complex and lengthy, analysis can lead in multiple directions, and it may be difficult to know when to stop analysis and start writing. This is particularly challenging in qualitative research because writing and analysis are often conducted simultaneously; however, insufficient analysis can stifle writing and frustrate the development of the results. When should writing the results then begin? In general a point is reached during data analysis where the findings become clear and fewer new insights are gained during analysis, although questions about the study findings may remain. This is a good point at which to begin to write because writing not only starts to clarify the findings even further but also uncovers areas that remain unclear and warrant further investigation in the data. At this point the circular process of writing and further analysis becomes most fruitful. During this time the core findings and main messages of the data also become clearer and the task of how to best report these findings begins.

Before beginning to write it is useful to have a "roadmap" of what to include in the results and the broad message of the study that will be presented. It is therefore useful to begin with an outline of the content of the results section, even though this may evolve during the writing process. This is particularly useful because focus group research can generate many study findings, but not all are included in the results or are relevant to the research objectives. It is also useful to take stock of all the writing that has been done thus far in the project, so as not to begin with a completely "blank page." There are likely to be multiple forms of preliminary results that can offer a starting point for writing the results, for example, interim reports to a sponsor, oral presentations, conference abstracts, or a whole array of analytic documents, such as early conceptualization of data and development of themes. Analytic memos may have been developed during data analysis, which highlight key findings, thoughts, and reflections, and provide useful points to begin to shape the results. Reviewing these outputs can provide a useful starting point to begin shaping the study results section.

It is important to make time for writing. Qualitative research takes considerably more time to write than other types of research, because of the process of simultaneous writing and further analysis to refine and verify emerging issues. Although this circular process in itself takes time, time is also needed to reflect deeply on data and how it informs the research problem. Good reflective writing simply takes time, which may not be valued if writing is perceived as simply recording an end product.

Developing an Argument

Study results are not presented in isolation. They are typically presented within a narrative or argument that takes the reader through the findings and indicates how each finding contributes to the overall message of the study. An argument offers a line of reasoning to make sense of the collective findings; it presents a perspective or develops an explanation for the phenomenon studied. An argument therefore provides the intellectual structure for the study results, within which the narrative descriptions of study findings and extracts of data are presented. A well-written results section offers a clear and coherent argument and uses the data well to support this underlying argument. Even when focus group research is used in mixed methods research, the findings still form one component of the research evidence that is used to construct an overall argument. In the beginning the writing may lack a clear argument that weaves the study findings together into a broader narrative or framework. Try to avoid writing study results like a descriptive "shopping list" of issues or the presentation of consecutive quotations with little narrative to guide the reader through the relevance of the issues to the overall research question.

There are many ways to construct an effective argument to present the study results. The most suitable type of argument to use is determined by the objectives of the study, the research question, and the nature of the study findings. Some examples of different types of arguments include the following.

Types of Arguments

A developmental argument	Used to explain how a social phenomenon develops (e.g., How do children become obese? What is the process of marriage migration?).
A mechanical argument	Used to explain how social phenomenon work (e.g., How do community gardens improve nutrition?).

A comparative argument	Used to compare different aspects of a phenomenon (e.g., Why are married women at greater risk of HIV transmission than single women? Why does unemployment cause greater stress in males than females?).
A causal argument	Used to explain why certain phenomena influence particular outcomes or occur in a specific context (e.g., How does delayed childbearing increase women's empowerment? Why is vitamin intake low despite free provision?).

An argument effectively embraces the study findings to convey the broader message of the study. An effective argument has several characteristics. First, an argument needs to be credible and convincing by using the study findings to demonstrate that the argument presented is the most plausible interpretation of the study findings. "Scholarly writers have to...express an argument clearly enough so that readers can follow the reasoning and accept the conclusions" (Becker, 1986, cited in Silverman, 2011b, p. 385). This involves not only presenting evidence to support the argument but also indicating why alternative explanations are implausible and addressing any contradictions in the study findings. Second, an argument should be systematic, by carefully demonstrating how the conclusions were developed and verified. This demonstrates the logic of how the conclusions were developed from the textual data and validated through rigorous data analysis. Third, an effective argument in qualitative research presents not only the central findings but also provides an indication of the variability and nuances within those findings. This provides the depth and richness expected of qualitative research findings. Fourth, it should be clear how the data presented in the argument were selected, what they represent, and how they are relevant to the overall argument presented. Data extracts need to be tightly woven into the argument and their contribution made clear, to avoid misinterpretation by readers. Overall, an effective argument in qualitative research needs to be transparent, so that readers not only understand the conclusions reached but also how these conclusions were arrived at, why they are plausible, and that they were based on thorough data analysis. For further reading on developing an argument see Mason (2002).

Structuring Narrative Accounts

The results of focus group research are often presented in narrative form and use quotations to exemplify issues. The results section can therefore be lengthy, detailed, and complex and readers can quickly become lost in the detail. An effective structure is therefore critical to help readers navigate the study findings and understand the central message of the study. A poor structure can obscure the study findings and their impact is then lost.

The first task in structuring a narrative account is to identify the key findings and the core message of the study. This can sometimes be the most challenging part. It involves identifying the main "story" of the data, the essential components of that story, and how to best tell the story. Although the study findings stem from rigorous data analysis, most focus group data are complex and reveal multiple findings, interrelationships, and cross-cutting themes. There may be multiple "storylines" or alternative outcomes for different subgroups of study participants, all of which increase the complexity of the results and add to the challenge of how to present them. It is easy to become overwhelmed by the volume and details of the data and lose sight of the central message of the study findings. It is important to remember that many details could be presented, but to remain focused on the most pertinent findings that respond to the research objectives.

It can also be useful to provide the reader with "signposts" to navigate the results section. For example, providing an overview paragraph that orients the reader to how the results are presented. This is particularly useful for focus group results, which may be presented in very different ways. Adding short sentences to indicate what is covered in each section, indicating how each section of the results contributes to the overall research problem, or using subheadings can assist readers to navigate a lengthy results section.

There are many ways to structure the results of focus group research. Some approaches are outlined next. Although this is not an exhaustive list, it provides a range of effective strategies to frame study findings. The most suitable structure to use is determined by the nature of the study findings and the purpose of the study.

Key Concepts

Focus group results may be structured by key concepts or themes. These are not the text-level codes that were used to code data during analysis, but higher level categories that are the product of data analysis. They may encompass a group of codes but represent a broader concept. Key concepts or themes may be used as subheadings followed by a descriptive narrative of each concept and how it contributes to an overall understanding of the study phenomenon. Using key concepts to structure the results reflects a higher level of abstraction from data, whereas the descriptive narrative or example quotations clearly link the findings back to the data.

An example of this structure is shown in a focus group study aimed at understanding the beliefs of diabetes prevention in the Bangladeshi community in the United Kingdom (Grace, Begum, Subhani, Kopelman, & Greenhalgh, 2008). This study used seven key concepts to structure the study results; some concepts included "responsibility" for diabetes prevention, which encompassed issues of control, faith, fear, and knowledge. Another concept was "structural constraints" to a healthy lifestyle, which included issues of time, money, childcare, safety language, and dietary choice. Each concept was used as a subheading in the results section and included a narrative description of the components of the concept using quotations to exemplify different issues. The study also included three types of study participants (lay people, religious leaders, and health professionals) whose perspectives on each concept were compared in the narrative descriptions. Another study by Sheu et al. (2012) presented focus group study findings by five key themes in relation to decision-making on renal replacement therapy. Each theme was used as a subheading in the results section, for example, "Theme Three: Poor awareness of alternative RRT options" and "Theme Five: family members' supportive involvement in RRT decisions." The description of each theme also included comparisons among the subgroups of the study participants (patients and family members; African Americans and non-African Americans).

Research Questions or Topics

Focus group results can be structured by research questions or topics. Research questions frame data collection and guide analysis, and can become a useful structure for presenting results. This structure involves presenting the question or topic discussed and then a synthesis of the issues identified. This is a useful structure when the research question presents distinct topics or when focus group data respond to a defined research question, as may be the case in mixed methods research. Where space is limited, results may be presented in table format, listing the question or topic with the range of responses, or example quotations included under each.

In a study of physician decision-making (O'Donnell, Lutfey, Marceau, & McKinlay, 2007) results were structured by five key questions that were asked in the focus group discussions. The results of each question were presented in table format that included the question asked and example quotations showing the range of responses by the two study populations of physicians in the United Kingdom and United States. This enables a summary of the focus group results to be gleaned from the table itself, including comparative differences between each group of physicians, whereas the narrative text provided a more detail description of the findings and a discussion of their implications. An example of one of the tables presented in this study is shown in Figure 4.1. The presentation of results in table format is optional, although a highly useful space-saving strategy.

Study results can also be structured by research questions but without the use of a summary table of results, as described in the previous example. Jette, Wilson, and Sparks (2007) conducted a focus group study on young womens' perceptions of smoking in popular films among smokers and nonsmokers. The study results were presented separately for smokers and nonsmokers and each section included results of two research questions: the effect of films on youths' smoking behavior and the impact of tobacco imagery on young viewers. The third research question identified differences in perception of smokers and nonsmokers. Using the research questions to structure the results can be a simple but effective presentation strategy for some focus group studies.

Population Subgroups
Focus group results can be structured by subgroups of the study population. This may involve presenting issues related to one subgroup followed by another, and is particularly effective for comparative research or where each subgroup presents different

---

Reasons to Participate in a Research Study

Question: 'What particular features of a research study would encourage you to participate?'

U.S Physicians	U.K General Practitioners
R: Being paid R: Who asked you and whether you're compensated R: And the virtue of the study. . . if you think it's going to accomplish something R: And not sell more pills, but it's going to really make you answer a very important question, and what you're saying is important, then I would think you'd find more people participating for nothing R: Doctors are highly motivated by a sense of professionalism and collegiality	R: The topic R: An angle to do with sort of improving health care. Improving medical practice, improving conditions of practice R: And here's a small amount of money for your time, I think that would buy more GPs than anything else, very sadly but it would. R: Ask to speak to the practice manager R: There's a thing about when you phone . . . R: You want to write the chairman of the primary group because they're the professional lead.

Figure 4.1. Presentation of focus group results by key questions. Reproduced with permission from "Using Focus Groups to Improve the Validity of Cross-National Survey Research: A Study of Physician Decision-Making," by A. O'Donnell, K. Lutfey, L. Marceau, and J. McKinlay, 2007, *Qualitative Health Research, 17(7)*, p. 971–981.

perspectives on the research issues, such as presenting results from different study sites (e.g., urban and rural) or different target populations (e.g., patients and clinicians). This structure is particularly effective for focus group research, which often comprises inbuilt subgroups where each focus group comprises participants of different socio-demographic backgrounds or characteristics. For example, focus group research in Lesotho, southern Africa, examined perceptions on the introduction of school sex education among school teachers, pupils, and parents, which provided an effective comparative structure to present the different issues and perspectives from the three subgroups of study participants (Mturi & Hennink, 2005).

Research Method

Where focus groups comprise a component of a mixed methods study, study results may be presented by each method of data collection. This may involve presenting the results of a quantitative method (e.g., a survey) followed by the focus group results, or vice versa. This structure is effective when each research method collects data on a different aspect of the research topic, for example a quantitative survey may collect sociodemographic data on the study population, whereas focus group discussions may collect data on specific topical issues. Alternatively, mixed methods research can be presented by topic thereby integrating the quantitative and qualitative findings for each topic (see later section on presenting mixed methods study results).

Typology

Study results may be presented as a typology that was developed during data analysis. A typology presents a categorization of phenomenon, such as different types of behaviors, perspectives, or outcomes. The results are then structured around a description of the categories that form the typology, using narrative or quotations to exemplify how each category is distinct. This is a more conceptual structure for presenting study results, therefore it can be useful to provide an example or brief case study of each "type" to balance the conceptual nature of a typology with tangible examples from the data.

Problem Solving

Focus group results may be presented in a problem-solving format, whereby the research problem is clearly stated and then study findings unroll a range of evidence-based solutions. This type of structure is effective where focus group data highlight a range of potential strategies or solutions to the research issues discussed.

Theory Development

Study results may be structured around describing how the findings contribute to the development of new theory or understanding of the phenomenon examined. In this structure focus group findings are used to present the empirical evidence for a new theory or explanation developed. Alternatively, study results may be presented to demonstrate how they "fit" or extend an existing theory, or how a theory can be made more culturally relevant to a certain study population. A conceptual diagram may visually depict the theory or phenomenon examined. Some examples are described next.

A focus group study by Woods-Giscombe (2010) aimed to develop a conceptual framework to understand the phenomenon of the "strong black woman/superwoman" and how it affects health and stress among African American women. The results section begins with the presentation of the conceptual framework (shown in Figure 4.2), which characterizes participants' perceptions of the superwoman role, their views on its development, and its perceived benefits and liabilities. The study results then follow this framework to describe in detail each component of the superwoman phenomenon, highlighting how perceptions of the phenomenon differ by age and education of participants from different focus groups. Throughout the narrative there is also a description of how the phenomenon of the superwoman influences health, particularly stress, among African American women.

In another study, Holmes, Winskell, Hennink, and Chidiac (2011) developed an empirical theory, using data from focus group discussions and in-depth interviews, to explain how the negative socio-economic cycle of HIV is reversed with microcredit. First, the negative economic cycle of HIV is described, whereby people with HIV have poor health and reduced work capacity, which reduces their economic resources so that they are unable to access treatment to improve their health. This negative cycle is perpetuated by the negative social perceptions of people with HIV, who are viewed as "living dead," an economic burden, and seen as noncontributing members of society. The study then developed an empirical theory that microcredit loans to people with HIV actually reverse this negative economic cycle, whereby microcredit loans provide capital that enables access to treatment, leading to improved health and increased work capacity. This positive economic cycle also changes the social perceptions of people living with HIV to be contributors to society, creditworthy, and seen as "cured." This theory was presented visually in two conceptual

What are the characteristics?
- Obligation to manifest strength
- Obligation to supress emotions
- Resistance to being vulnerable or dependent
- Determination to succeed, despite limited resources
- Obligation to help others

What are the contributing contextual factors?
- Historical legacy of racial or gender stereotyping or oppression
- Lessons from foremothers
- Past history of disappointment, mistreatment or abuse
- Spiritual values

What are perceived benefits?
- Preservation of self/survival
- Preservation of African American community
- Preservation of African American family

What are the perceived liabilities?
- Strain in interpersonal (e.g. romantic) relationships
- Stress-related health behaviors (e.g. postponement of self-care, emotional eating, poor sleep)
- Embodiment of stress (e.g. anxiety, depressive symptoms, adverse maternal health)

Figure 4.2. Conceptual framework of the "strong black woman/superwoman" phenomenon. Reproduced with permission from "Superwoman Schema: African American Women's Views on Stress, Strength and Health," by C. Woods-Giscombe, 2010, *Qualitative Health Research, 20(5)*, p. 668–683.

diagrams (shown in Figure 4.3) showing the negative and positive socio-economic cycle of HIV and microcredit.

Chronology

Focus group results may be structured as a chronology, a process, or as stages of an event. This involves first distinguishing each stage of a chronology and then describing the issues or influences at each stage. For example, focus group research among young people in Pakistan used a chronology of life events from puberty to marriage to present the study findings on knowledge acquisition about sexual health, which differed distinctly at various life stages (see Figure 4.4). This chronologic structure allowed a comparison of knowledge acquisition by gender at each life stage (Hennink, Rana, & Iqbal, 2005).

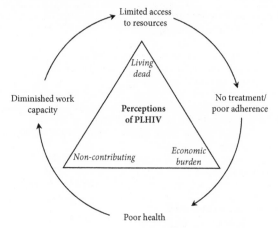

Negative socio-economic HIV/AIDS cycle

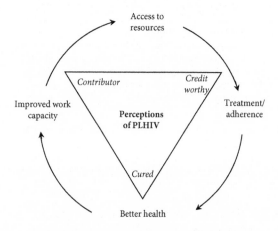

Positive socio-economic HIV/AIDS cycle

Figure 4.3. Visual presentation of theory development. Reproduced with permission from K. Holmes, K. Winskell, M. Hennink, and S. Chidiac, "Microfinance and HIV Mitigation among People Living With HIV in the Era of Anti-Retroviral Therapy: Emerging Lessons from Cote d'Ivoire," 2011, *Global Public Health, 6*, p. 458.

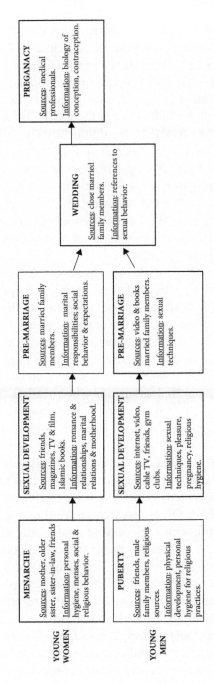

Figure 4.4. Process of knowledge acquisition on sexual development among young people in Pakistan. Adapted and reprinted with permission from M. Hennink, I. Rana, and R. Iqbal, "Knowledge of Personal and Sexual Development amongst Young People in Pakistan," 2005, *Culture, Health and Sexuality, 7(4)*, p. 319–332.

Using Quotations

Perhaps the most common form of reporting focus group research is to include verbatim quotations of participants' words to highlight issues described. The textual narrative of the report typically provides a synthesis of the issues, whereas quotations provide the richness and detail of participants' own words. Quotations therefore provide "a direct link between the more abstract content of the results and the actual data; in addition, they are also the strongest connection between the reader and the voices of the original participants" (Morgan, 2010, p. 718). Quotations can also convey more subtle information, such as emotions or reactions of participants to the issues discussed. These details can be lost in a strictly textual description of the issues. Presenting quotations therefore has strong benefits and remains a long-standing tradition of reporting qualitative research.

The use of quotations is also seen as a tool to validate the issues reported, to demonstrate that they were indeed present in the data. Quotations provide tangible examples of participant's words and expressions. However, the use of quotations as a tool to assess validity of the research findings can lead readers and reviewers to expect quotations in all qualitative reports as a validity check for the issues reported. Qualitative research can therefore be criticized for making unsupported assertions when readers do not see a quotation to support each issue presented. Although it is possible to present quotations for explicit issues, for others the presentation of quotations is not possible. For example, some issues may be well grounded in data but the evidence is spread throughout the data, so there may be no explicit quotation that highlights the issue clearly or succinctly enough to include in the report (Corden & Sainsbury, 1996). Other research findings may be more conceptual, presenting concepts derived analytically and although well evidenced by the data the presentation of a quotation is not possible. In these situations, the lack of quotations should not detract from the validity of the concepts described. The expectation of quotations as the only evidence that results are empirically grounded is unfortunate. This situation can corral qualitative researchers into presenting simple descriptive results using quotations as evidence, whereas studies using qualitative data to develop theory or more conceptual explanations are not given the credit deserved. There are multiple ways to demonstrate validity of the study findings aside from the presentation of quotations. These are discussed in the section on grounding study findings and in Chapter 5.

It is tempting to fill the results section with data extracts. However, consider the reasons for including quotations and use them judiciously so they make a clear contribution to the study results. Quotations should have a clear purpose and support the narrative argument presented in the report. Effective quotations add value to the results presented; however, if a quotation conveys no more than can be stated in the narrative text there is little benefit in its inclusion. For example, a quotation stating "the services are expensive for us" contributes little that cannot simply be stated in the text. An alternative quotation stating "the service is so expensive it will take a whole month of my salary just to pay the consultation fee" conveys more detail on the magnitude of the issue and its impact on a participant. Quotations can also be used to convey more subtle information than the words themselves, such as conveying emotions or language used by participants, thereby providing greater detail on the issue being reported.

The number of quotations to use is determined by their purpose. For example, one quotation may be sufficient to show a typical response to an issue, two quotations may be used to compare different stances on an issue, whereas a series of quotations can demonstrate a range of issues in the data. Avoid the temptation to use too many quotations because this quickly diminishes their effect, and can swamp readers with data that detracts from the main message of the results. Ritchie and Lewis (2003, p. 290) state that "the overuse of cited passages can make a research account tedious to read, voluminous in length and easily distract from the clarity of the main commentary." Careful consideration of the purpose of each quotation reduces their overuse in the study results.

Consider how quotations are selected to avoid presenting overly vivid extracts that may provide an imbalanced perspective of the issues. Bogdan and Taylor (1975, p. 145) suggest that "you should resist the temptation to overuse certain colourful materials at the expense of others. If you cannot find an alternative example, the point you are trying to make may not be as important as thought originally."

It is also useful to check the balance between narrative text and quotations. The narrative text should provide a clear argument or structure to guide the reader through the study findings, with quotations used to illustrate the issues and provide contextual detail. Therefore, the text essentially reports the outcome of data analyses, whereas quotations represent the raw data. If too much of the results section is taken up with quotations and little narrative text, it equates to presenting the reader with unprocessed data. This suggests that little effort has been given to data analysis and interpretation. Therefore, quotations should be used thoughtfully and embedded within the broader descriptive text rather than replacing the text.

Some guidelines for selecting and using quotations are provided next, as adapted from Hennink, Hutter, and Bailey (2011, p. 281).

Guidelines for Using Quotations

Type	Is a quotation from an individual participant most appropriate? Is an extract of group interaction relevant? How can interactive dialogue be included?
Purpose	What is the purpose of the quotation? (e.g., typical view, contrasting views) What issue does the quotation highlight? Does it add value to the text or duplicate it?
Clarity	Is the issue clear from the quotation? Can editing improve the clarity of the quotation? Should the moderator's question be included?
Relevance	Is the quotation relevant to the argument made in the text? Does the quotation add value to the results?
Balance	Is there a balance of narrative text versus quotations? Are the quotations effectively embedded in an argument? Do the quotations exemplify the text or replace it?

Length	Is the quotation long enough to provide context to the issue highlighted? Is the quotation too long?
Number	How many quotations are included for the same issue? How many quotations are in the entire report? What is the justification for including each quotation?
Selection	How was the quotation selected? Can alternative quotations be found for the issue?
Reference	How is the quotation referenced to the data? Can attribution add to the clarity of the quotation? (e.g., "unmarried men's group," "rural women")
Ethics	Is the quotation anonymous? Can the participant be identified from the quotation?

Data extracts are sometimes edited to reduce their length and improve readability. Textual data reflects participants' natural speech, which may comprise incomplete thoughts, repetition, pauses, rambling statements, or interruptions by other participants. Quotations may be presented exactly as they were spoken or edited to improve the readability or clarity of the point being made; however, any changes should not alter the meaning of the original comment. Editing may involve removing sections of speech not related to the issue being reported or adding words to complete the logic of a comment. Missing text is often replaced by ellipses, such as (...), and added words included inside square brackets. Other edits may be made to maintain confidentiality. Rubin and Rubin (2005, p. 262) state that "as long as the meaning is preserved, the words that are quoted were actually said, and you mark the places where you made omissions, this practice is acceptable." The example below shows edits to the original text to improve clarity, while indicating where changes have been made with ellipses and square brackets.

Original text: "I can tell you about that place. They just shout at us, like we are illiterates, yes, it happens, my daughter was there for her pregnancy, it was her fourth child she was knowledgeable but, they didn't, even her child was there with her. It's a terrible service, you leave feeling worse than when you arrived!"

Edited text: "[Nurses] just shout at us, like we are illiterates...It's a terrible service, you leave feeling worse than when you arrived!"

Providing attribution to quotations helps readers to better interpret a comment. Attribution involves indicating the characteristics of the focus group from which the quotation was taken, such as certain sociodemographic characteristics of the group (e.g., gender, age range, ethnicity, and so forth) or details of the study sites (e.g., rural or urban). Attribution can be included after a quotation, such as "(unmarried males)" or "(rural women's group)." Alternatively, attribution may be embedded in the sentence before the quotations, such as "The following extract from the discussion among unmarried males in the rural study site illustrates the importance of marriage." Attribution is important because it provides context about the quotation as the meaning of a comment can differ depending on the characteristics of the speaker. For example, the quotation "Vaccinations for children should be the choice of the parents alone" is interpreted differently if the speaker is a parent or a medical provider. In addition, attribution can indicate that quotations were selected from a range of focus group discussions to indicate the pervasiveness of an issue across the data, thus also indicating analytic rigor. Attribution is particularly useful when comparing comments from different types of focus group discussions, such as men and women's groups or rural and urban groups.

Reporting Group Interaction

Focus group data provide a unique opportunity to present interaction among participants, which can add additional insight to the issues reported. During a focus group discussion participants present ideas, exchange views, and react to the comments of others; there may be rapid exchanges as they debate issues or multiple comments can show consensus on an issue. This type of interaction is critical for generating focus group data, and is encouraged by a moderator and by the design of the questions asked. Focus group data therefore inherently include interaction and provide an opportunity to report exchanges between participants that are not available in data from in-depth interviews. However, group interaction is rarely reported in focus group research. A review of studies using focus group discussions published between 1946 and 1996 found that focus group data are most frequently presented as quotations from individuals with interactions among participants rarely reported or shown (Wilkinson, 1998), thereby seeming as if there was no interaction. Group interaction has therefore been described as a source of data that is underused and under-reported in focus group research (Duggleby, 2005).

There are two broad approaches to analyzing, and thus reporting, focus group interaction. For some studies, the focus of analysis is on *how* participants discuss issues in a group discussion, whereas for others the focus is on the substantive content of *what* is said in the discussion (Morgan, 2010). Researchers focusing on how participants talk are clearly most interested in examining the interactive exchanges among participants, using analytic approaches, such as conversation analysis, discourse analysis, and others. In this type of research the interaction among participants becomes the data that are analyzed and the focus of analysis is on the nature of the interactions. These studies are most likely to present and discuss interaction among participants in reporting focus group findings. In contrast, researchers interested in the substantive content of the group discussion focus almost exclusively on the issues discussed, which requires little attention to the interactive component of the discussion. These studies typically report the issues themselves, often presenting quotations from individual participants to reflect these issues. The interactive discussion from which the issues arose is not the focus of the analysis and is therefore seldom reflected in reporting the findings. This is entirely appropriate for the goals of reporting substantive issues. However, even in substantive research there are situations where reflecting interaction can add richness to the data presented and additional insight to the research findings. Group interaction may be reported implicitly or explicitly in substantive research as described next. The following suggestions are drawn primarily from Morgan (2010) and Duggleby (2005).

Interaction among focus group participants may be implied when presenting quotations from individual participants, even though it is not reported directly. Reporting an interactive exchange between participants can add considerable length to a research report. Therefore, quotations from an individual participant may be used to sum up a discussion or to present a "typical" comment from the discussion of an issue, without reporting the actual interactive discussion. This enables the length of the research report to be managed yet still implicitly suggest that interaction occurred. Alternatively, a series of quotations from individuals may be presented to identify the range of issues discussed on a topic, rather than presenting the actual interactive exchange on this topic. These strategies do not report or describe interaction per se but implicitly suggest interaction occurred during the group discussion.

There are four approaches to report interaction more explicitly. The first two approaches involve describing interaction in a narrative paragraph using "lead-in" or "follow-out" text, and then presenting a single illustrative quotation from the discussion. The third approach involves directly presenting an extract of interactive dialogue among several participants on an issue. A fourth approach uses text as a joiner between quotations to reflect group interaction.

The first approach to reporting group interaction is to use a "lead-in." A "lead-in" is a brief paragraph that describes the nature of the group discussion on a specific issue, before including a single illustrative quotation of the issue. This strategy reflects group interaction on the issue without including lengthy segments of interactive dialogue. A "lead-in" can provide useful context about the group's interaction on the issue, for example if the issue was discussed with reluctance, or led to a heated debate, whether it was a lengthy discussion, if there was consensus or divided perspectives on the issue. By providing this descriptive context about the discussion only an illustrative quotation is then needed to exemplify the issue. A "lead-in" can therefore summarize the group interaction more concisely than including an extract of the interactive discussion in the results. The following example shows a "lead-in" paragraph before a quotation that conveys the nature of the group interaction (validating, affirmative); the receptive group environment; and indicates unspoken aspects of communication within the group, such as laughter, humor, and head shaking.

The first group member to do so in each case was met with validating statements such as, 'Yes, to me, too, it happened.' Group laughter and affirmative head shaking formed the receptive environment in which additional personal revelation were made by group members. Humor seemed to ease the conversation, as in the way this woman described her husband's behavior when she had first fallen ill:

I was so thin he didn't even want to look at me. Even to look at me, when he goes out at night and comes back, when he finds me sleeping. 'Move. Let me sleep! Let me sleep! Are you still alive!' [The women laugh]. 'I am alive. You thought I was dead when my time has not yet come? When my time comes, you will hear of it on the road—'your wife is gone. But right now I am still around.' I was suffering alone with my children... (Mkandawire-Valhmu & Stevens, 2010, p. 689)

A "follow-out" is a second approach to reporting group interaction, which is the reverse of the "lead-in" approach. A "follow-out" provides interpretive comment about the nature of the group discussion after presenting a single quotation, thereby extending the context of interaction after a quotation. "Follow-out" text after a quotation may indicate the commonality of the issue expressed in the quotation, what followed from the discussion of this topic, what was concluded from the period of discussion, reactions of participants to a comment, and so forth. The example below is taken from an article about the influence of popular film on young people's smoking behavior (Jette et al., 2007). It shows a "follow-out" paragraph after a quotation that provides interpretive comment on the two reasons influencing the issue described in the quotation that were reflected in the broader discussion of the issue. This example also includes a brief "lead-in" sentence to indicate that this was an issue raised by participants.

Members in one of the groups discussed the possibility that smoking in films by a favorite actor might influence young people to start to smoke. As one participant explained,

And if they like... the character, or whatever, and they kind of relate to the character, then it makes it more like, 'oh well,

I can be like her in that movie. Oh, I look just like her, like, or him.' Right? So, it does kind of influence, but you don't like to say it. Like, you don't like to actually think you're doing it because that person is doing it? But it does kind of, like in a subtle way.

Embedded in the last comment are two insights into why young people might deny that movies might influence their smoking uptake. The first is that the influence is so subtle that they are not aware of it. The second is that young people (and people in general) do not like to admit that they are influenced by the mass media, as is suggested by the comment, "You don't like to actually think you're doing it because that person is doing it" (Jette et al., 2007, p. 330).

The "lead-in" and "follow-out" are simple strategies for reflecting group interactions when reporting focus group data that add depth and context to reporting the study results. They embed interaction within the body of the text itself, providing brevity and depth to the study results. They also allow greater insight into the nature of the interactive discussion on specific issues, which provides an additional lens through which to report the research issues. Both approaches can also be used together. The following example is taken from an article about women living with HIV in Malawi (Mkandawire-Valhmu & Stevens, 2010). It demonstrates the use of a "lead-in" and "follow-out" strategy, whereby the "lead-in" text is used to describe the nature of group interaction around the topic of stigma, such as agreement about stigma among participants; the language used (the collective *we*); and the commonality of the issue. A single exemplary quotation is then presented, followed by a "follow-out" paragraph that describes participants reactions (laughter, recognition, affirmation), and indicates that the discussion continued on the topic.

As women agreed with each other about the frequency of such circumstances and explained their actions, they build consensus about what stigma meant to them as women living with HIV and about how best to respond to it. The collective *we* was frequently used in their explanations and responses to each other. For instance, in the following excerpt a woman characterized the gossip spread in her village:

They just whisper about us. 'Have you seen those with AIDS? They are not going to complete this year. When they start taking that medicine, they get fat. They just die, those that have AIDS!' But we feel, as long as we know our future, as long as we are taking medications—'You go ahead and laugh at us.'

Women laughed with recognition and affirmation of this circumstance, quickly following with similar accounts. After agreeing that she had endured similar humiliations one woman detailed her interpretation...(Mkandawire-Valhmu & Stevens, 2010, p. 688)

A third approach to reporting focus group interaction involves directly presenting segments of interactive discussion in the research report. This format presents the reader directly with the context of the group discussion and can convey additional information about how an issue was discussed by participants. For example, a segment of interactive discussion may highlight a range of perspectives on an issue indicating broad diversity, whereas short rapid responses may indicate an issue is highly charged; or a range of similar comments in the dialogue may indicate a broad consensus among participants about an issue. Presenting excerpts of interaction can have clear benefits. The challenge is to balance the often lengthy sections of interactive discussion with the word limits of typical journal articles. Morgan (2010) suggests that when faced with the choice of presenting a segment of interactive discussion versus a comment from one participant, where both are similar in length and impact, presenting interaction is preferable because it connects the reader directly with the dynamics of the group discussion in which the issue was discussed. An additional benefit of showing interaction is to demonstrate how group participants coconstruct meaning around the research issues during the discussion (Wilkinson, 1998; Duggleby, 2005), which may be relevant to some research goals.

The following example is taken from the same focus group study described previously on the influence of popular film on young people's smoking behavior. It shows how interactive dialogue among participants is reported to exemplify how scenes in a film resonated with participants real life experiences of smoking. The direct presentation of group interaction is beneficial here because it demonstrates consensus among participants on this issue.

> Often, discussion with smokers about the believability of a clip segued into conversations about 'real life' smoking, as the participants drew on personal experiences with cigarettes and compared the smoking depiction in the movie clip to their life. The following represent typical responses:
>
> Speaker 1: She [Julia Roberts] knew that she wasn't allowed to smoke in there, but she didn't care because she was upset or whatever...Because when you are stressed, the first thing you go for, if you're a smoker, is your smokes...
>
> Speaker 2: This morning.
>
> Speaker 1: Yeah, like after a bad test.
>
> Speaker 3: If you're in a bad mood, then you need a smoke. (Jette et al., 2007, p. 331)

Presenting quotations of interactive dialogue is also beneficial to demonstrate short "lightning strike" responses on an issue. For example, the following extract shows an interactive exchange about name-calling toward people who are on antiretroviral medication for HIV in Malawi. Presenting the actual interactive exchange in the study results demonstrates the shared experiences of public humiliation among participants, who were HIV-positive women, and the sense in which this issue was discussed, with laughter. The following extract shows the name-calling the women experienced.

Participant 1: 'You're eating ARVs [antiretroviral medication]!' they say.

Participant 2: 'Aren't you eating ARVs?' 'Those who eat ARVs!'

Participant 1: Our name becomes 'Those who eat ARVs'

Participant 3: 'Have you seen the one on ARVs?'

Participant 1: 'She lives a life of ARVs' When you are passing by you hear, 'Look at the one on ARVs' [The women laugh]. (Mkandawire-Valhmu & Stevens, 2010, p. 690)

A fourth approach to reflecting group interaction is to separate the presentation of quotations with a sentence to reflect the interactive discussion that took place. For example, after the presentation of one quotation and leading into a second quotation use a sentence such as the following:

'Another woman followed with...'
'Another participant reinforced this collective experience of...'
'This was quickly followed by similar accounts...'
'The group interaction continued with another woman agreeing that...'
'Others in the group responded with empathy...'

Alternatively, after the presentation of a quotation indicate the general response of others, for example [several women, in agreement, say 'Yes, it's true.'] or [most participants nodded in agreement with the speaker].

These examples show different approaches to reflect interaction in reporting focus group results. Consideration is needed on which format is most suitable for presenting data extracts from focus group data, whether to present actual segments of interactive discussion versus an illustrative quotation with a "lead-in" or "follow-out" narrative paragraph about the nature of the interaction. The purpose of presenting each type of data extract needs to be clear for the reader and contribute to the overall argument presented in the study results.

Visual Presentation of Results

Narrative description of study findings forms the foundation of many focus group reports. However, study findings can also be effectively presented in visual formats, which can range from a structured list of issues to a flow chart or a more elaborate conceptual diagram. Visual presentation of focus group results can simplify a complex process, display core linkages between components of data, or summarize a key message, thereby making the study findings more accessible to readers. Whether or not a diagram is appropriate depends entirely on the type of results being presented and whether these lend themselves to a visual presentation format. In general, diagrams are most effective when used sparingly. They should be simple and easy to follow and need to be explained in the textual narrative of the results, because few diagrams are completely self-explanatory.

Using visual displays to communicate focus group results has multiple benefits. A diagram can assist in data reduction because it essentially summarizes information that may otherwise need several pages of descriptive text. Visual displays reduce long textual descriptions of the study findings; however, some explanation of a diagram is always required to ensure its correct interpretation by readers. Visual displays can also simplify the presentation of complex relationships because they can show different dimensions and levels and the relationships between these, which provides the reader with an immediate summary of the research findings from which to better understand the narrative text. Visual presentation of data can also convey depth of the research findings by displaying the range and diversity of study issues, for example by presenting a typology of issues or a concept map of key components of the study results. For example, a study by Wong, Sands, and Solomon (2010) aimed to conceptualize perceptions of "community" among users of mental health services. The authors presented the results of the study in a concept map, which displayed the four types of communities identified by study participants (their cultural identity community, treatment community, faith community, and neighborhood community) and a range of domains depicting the needs that each type of community fulfills. The diagram showed that some domains were common to all communities, whereas others were specific to a single community. Overall the concept map provided a visual display of the components of data and the linkages between them, which were then described in the text with example quotations. Finally, visual displays of study findings can also break up a qualitative research report, which is typically long and textually dense. In another study, Humbert et al. (2006) summarized the key findings of focus group research in a table using an ecologic framework (see Figure 4.5), whereby results were presented at three levels (intra-personal, social, and environmental influences on physical activity) and two columns were used to compare results by high and low socio-economic status of participants. This provides the reader with a quick snapshot of the overall findings, which were then described in the narrative text with example quotations.

Factor	High Socioeconomic Status	Low Socioeconomic Status
Intrapersonal	Time barriers: work, homework, other scheduled activities (e.g. piano Fun: perceived competence, perceived skill	Time barriers: family obligations, homework Fun: perceived competence, perceived skill
Social	Friends Parental involvement	Friends Adult involvement
Environmental	Type of activity: seasonal programming, diverse choices	Proximity Cost Facilities Safety

Figure 4.5. Presentation of focus group results using an ecological framework and socioeconomic status. Reproduced with permission from M. Humbert, et al., "Factors that Influence Physical Activity Participation among High- and Low-SES Youth," 2006, *Qualitative Health Research, 16(4)*, p. 467–483.

Developing visual displays of focus group results may begin while writing study results or even earlier during data analysis. The process of analyzing data may have produced a working diagram to understand emerging issues, such as the sketch of a timeline, a grouping of issues, or an elementary flow chart. These early sketches may have been used as tools for conceptualizing data during analysis but they can often be further developed and become effective formats for presenting the results in the final report. Therefore, it is worth revisiting working documents of data analysis to spur ideas for presenting focus group results visually. A study report may include several diagrams, such as a list of issues and a more elaborate conceptual framework; however, the overuse of diagrams begins to diminish their effect. There are endless possibilities for visual presentation of study findings, some possibilities are described next.

A *structured list* can bring together seemingly diverse issues from a group discussion under logical topics. A list of issues may also be ranked, grouped, or simply highlight characteristics of a phenomenon.

A *flowchart* can highlight a distinct process, by showing discrete stages, or the sequence of events. This may take the form of a timeline, lifecycle, or pathway diagram.

An *inductive model* is a conceptual framework that describes or explains the study phenomenon. It demonstrates how the study findings link together to understand the research problem more conceptually and is usually presented as a diagram (examples are seen in Figures 1.2, 4.3, and 4.4).

A *theoretical framework* may present how the study findings developed a theoretical framework or extended or modified an existing theory, perhaps by developing new explanations or concepts, or adapting it for a specific population subgroup (Figure 4.2 is an example).

Reporting Numbers

It may be unclear whether focus group research findings can be presented numerically in addition to narrative text. Qualitative research is typically presented as narrative text, which may include descriptions of the study issues, narrative case studies, or quotations from study participants. However, some journal reviewers or editors feel compelled to encourage researchers to report qualitative data in numerical terms, by indicating the frequency or distribution of issues in the study population, as is usual for quantitative data.

Reporting qualitative data in numerical terms can be inappropriate for several reasons. First, using numerical terms, such as frequencies or percentages, to report qualitative findings can be misleading because it suggests to readers that data are representative and therefore study results are generalizable. Second, and more importantly, reporting study findings in numerical terms simply fails to embrace the benefits of qualitative research, which is to describe the characteristics of issues, explain phenomenon, and understand contextual influences on complex social phenomenon rather than to represent findings numerically. Reducing qualitative findings to a number simply neglects these benefits. In addition, quantifying results from focus group discussions may be ineffective because the unit of data collection is the group, so only the number of groups reporting an issue could potentially be quantified and this may provide little insight on the issues examined.

Instead, reporting how issues are distributed within focus group data can be achieved in descriptive ways, thereby avoiding misrepresenting the data by using numerical measures. For example, use descriptive words (e.g., many, most, few) to highlight whether an issue is common or rarely mentioned, which indicates pervasiveness of issues without using numerical measures that suggest statistical prevalence. Focus on describing the issues themselves by examining their context, meaning, and influences, rather than reporting the number of participants who reported those issues. Describe the variation in issues raised, different perspectives on those issues, or categories of responses to identify patterns in data or to explain issues. These approaches to reporting focus group data reflect the qualitative tradition in which data were collected and capitalize on the strengths of this approach, rather than attempting to report issues in numerical terms.

This is not to say that simple counting is not used at all in focus group research. Making a tally of certain issues is often used as an analytic tool in qualitative research to identify patterns and identify issues that are more or less common. However, these tally counts are usually not reported in the study results. Focus group data present challenges for such simple counting of issues, however, because not every participant responds to each issue discussed. Therefore, presenting a descriptive narrative of the issues from focus group data is more appropriate.

Reflecting Context in Results

All social phenomenon need to be understood in context; however, reporting context can sometimes be overlooked. Many types of contexts can be reported in focus group research, such as the personal context of the moderator, the sociocultural context of the study population, the physical context of the study site, the broader political or historical context that shaped the research issues, or the methodological context in which data were collected. These aspects of context are often reported in the background or methods section of the report (see Chapter 3), but can also be reflected in the study results.

Contextual influences often shape the phenomenon studied in focus group research and therefore it is important to include different aspects of context in reporting study results. Using quotations from study participants is a common strategy to convey context in the study results. A verbatim quotation can convey a great deal of contextual information. Quotations not only help to present the research issues in the words of the study participants, but also communicate expressions used by participants and the emotion with which issues are conveyed, which can have a greater impact on a reader than simply describing the issues in narrative form. For example, the results section may indicate that the main barrier to using a service was its cost; however, a quotation may state, "Of course we would like to use it, but it's the cost, it's too expensive. Most of the people here are unemployed, how can we afford it? We would have to decide either to pay for food or go to the clinic, it's that simple." This short quotation conveys not only that cost is a barrier to service use, but also the social context of unemployment, the widespread nature of this issue among study participants, and the trade-offs needed to use the service because of its cost. Therefore, well-chosen quotations can provide very powerful examples of context and add richness to focus group results.

Reporting quotations can also reflect the methodological context in which data were collected. Including a segment of dialogue among focus group participants not only presents the issues raised but also conveys the group context in which the issues were discussed. Similarly, it can be useful to include the moderator's question or prompt before a participant's comment to reflect the qualitative context of data collection and provide greater insight into the comment made. Furthermore, identifying the characteristics of the focus group participants after a quotation also reflects the context of the speakers. This can be done by including attribution after a quotation, such as "unemployed men's group." Attribution provides contextual information about the study participants, which helps to interpret a quotation. For example, a comment on the importance of breastfeeding is interpreted differently if spoken by breastfeeding mothers versus medical providers. Therefore, identifying who is speaking provides additional context to a quotation that helps readers to interpret the comment.

Contextual detail can also be included in the descriptive narrative of issues in the results section. Providing descriptive depth about the study results provides rich contextual information that is a hallmark of qualitative research. In reporting study results, examine whether the descriptive narrative provides sufficient contextual information to understand the issue, highlight its context within the study findings by indicating if the issue is central or peripheral in the study findings, and describe variation within the issue itself by including any nuances around the issue. For example, if travel time is reported as problematic, do the physical road conditions in the research sites or the lack of public transport in the area need to be described? Providing descriptive depth enables the study findings to be interpreted in the relevant context. Including photographs can be another way to convey context visually, particularly the physical context of the study location. However, ethical issues need to be considered whenever presenting photographs.

Reporting reflexivity in the study findings, where appropriate, can also provide contextual information on whether characteristics of the research team may have influenced a particular study finding. At times a focus group moderator may share personal information with study participants that may have influenced what participants share in the group discussion. This is worth reporting in the study findings, because it influences how a finding may be interpreted.

Finally, in making recommendations from the study findings, it is important to place these within the appropriate context. This may involve, for example, highlighting the social or cultural context of the study participants, the broader political context, or the economic context of an institution or social setting. For example, it is futile to recommend that women use contraception to reduce fertility in socially conservative contexts where women are not afforded such decision-making power or the social context is such that high fertility is desired. Therefore, recommendations need to be contextually relevant, feasible, and evidence based.

Grounding the Results

Focus group research can be criticized for making seemingly unsupported assertions when reporting study findings. Even though the study findings presented may be the outcome of rigorous data analysis, it is still necessary to demonstrate how the findings were "grounded," or well supported by data. Grounding study findings means demonstrating that findings emerged from data, that they are indeed supported by data, and that the explanations or arguments developed actually fit the data. Demonstrating how study findings are grounded is typically described in the methods section of the research report, but is also necessary in reporting the study results. This deflects any criticism that findings presented are unsupported by data and therefore a result of interpretation bias.

In the methods section it is important to describe the analytic procedures used to ground study findings. A range of strategies may have been applied during data analysis to ensure that findings reported, concepts developed, and explanations or theories presented were empirically supported. For example, an issue may have been validated by its constant repetition throughout the data, a concept may be validated as it encompasses a range of well-grounded themes, whereas an explanation may have been validated through participant feedback meetings. There are many strategies for grounding study findings relevant to the analytic approach used. What is important is that these are explicitly described in the research methods.

The results section needs to reflect the strategies used to validate the study findings. Some strategies for grounding study findings are simply conducted as analytic tasks and stated in the study methods, whereas other strategies for grounding study findings can be reflected in the way the study findings are presented or described. Three writing strategies can be used to demonstrate that study findings are well grounded. First, demonstrate that each component of data reported is grounded in the data itself or how it was validated. For example, using in vivo terms (from participants own words) when describing an issue demonstrates that it originated from participants own words, stating that a particular issue was repeatedly mentioned throughout the data shows it is well supported, or when describing a concept highlight the specific issues that contributed to the development of that concept. These strategies can concisely demonstrate how different components of the results are evidenced in data and thus well grounded. Second, show how the argument or theory presented fits the study data, which implicitly demonstrates that it is well supported by the study data. Showing the fit of interpretations demonstrates the robustness of the argument or theory and convinces a reader that what is presented is plausible and supported by data. This involves not only presenting evidence to support the stance described but also involves showing why the data do not support alternative explanations. Describing the absence of alternative explanations or presenting data that explicitly refute alternative views is a strong indicator that the explanations proposed actually fit the study data. Finally, show the nuances or limitations of the study findings, to demonstrate how data were used to refine study results. Describe the nuances found in issues presented, or whether some findings relate only to a sub-group of study participants, or the conditions under which certain findings are valid. These details provide contextual detail to demonstrate how each issue is shaped and supported by the study data.

Transferability of Results

In writing the results of focus group research, there is an inevitable question about whether results are relevant outside of the specific context in which the study was conducted. This is referred to as "generalizability" in quantitative research, which is somewhat problematic to apply directly to qualitative research; therefore, the term "transferability" is often used instead. Transferability refers to the wider relevance of qualitative study findings and their applicability to other contexts, without being generalizable in a statistical sense. The transferability of study results is typically addressed in the results or discussion sections of an academic report. Although some results of qualitative research are not transferable, much qualitative research does have resonance outside the specific context of the study. In the study results, it is important to note how the study results may be relevant to other contexts. This involves outlining the nature and context in which the study findings may be transferable. Ritchie and Lewis (2003) describe three forms in which qualitative research findings may be considered as transferable. They suggest considering (1) whether the issues and concepts reported are reflective of those found in a larger parent population (i.e., representation); (2) whether study findings can be applied to other contexts outside the study itself (i.e., inference); and (3) whether results contribute to development or refinement of empirical theory (i.e., theoretical relevance). Each of these is described more fully in Chapter 5. In writing and interpreting study findings it is important to clarify for the reader the type of transferability that is applicable; the context in which results may be transferable; and the validity of transferability (i.e., why the study results can be applied more broadly).

Presenting Mixed Methods Study Results

Focus group discussions are commonly used in mixed methods research, either with quantitative methods (e.g., a survey) or with other qualitative methods (e.g., in-depth interviews or observation). A mixed methods research design enables the research issue to be examined from different perspectives, thereby providing more comprehensive understanding of the issue than using a single approach. However, qualitative and quantitative research generate very different data, which cannot simply be woven together without an acknowledgment of their differences. One of the challenges in presenting the results of mixed methods research is to identify the most effective strategy to present the different types of research results.

The study design, the purpose of each method of data collection, and the nature of the study findings all influence how to present the results of mixed methods research. Data from each method of data collection first need to be analyzed according to procedures appropriate to the research paradigm in which the data were collected. Qualitative data need to be analyzed by following procedures of the interpretive paradigm, whereas quantitative data are analyzed in the positivist paradigm (see Chapter 2 for more on research paradigms). After the study findings from each method of data collection have been generated, the most effective method to present the study results to meet the research objectives can be determined.

One of the first decisions is which type of data will lead the study findings. Will the focus group data shape the main story of the research with quantitative data used to supplement this, or will the quantitative findings shape the structure of the study findings with extracts from the focus group discussions used to provide contextual evidence? One drawback of the latter approach is that qualitative research is often only used to provide illustrative quotations rather than being used to its full potential in providing contextual explanations and identifying variation and nuances in the study findings.

A subsequent decision is whether to integrate or separate the findings from mixed methods research. Integrating study findings is possible where each method of data collection covered similar topics or issues, whereby the results may be presented by topic, integrating relevant findings from each type of data. For example, results of survey data may present the prevalence of certain behavior, whereas focus group data are used to describe the context of that behavior. One of the challenges of integrating study findings in this way is that qualitative methods generate much more data, therefore requiring succinct presentation of study findings. A further issue arises when the findings from different research methods present contradictory findings on the same issue. In this case the reasons for the discrepancy should be explored and, if possible, explained. If the discrepancy remains unexplained, such as when there is insufficient data to explore it further, this should then be noted in the study findings for further examination in future research.

An alternative strategy for presenting findings from mixed methods research is to present findings from each method of data collection separately, such as presenting quantitative research findings followed by qualitative findings, or vice versa. This strategy is appropriate when the issues from each method of data collection do not overlap, and so cannot be integrated by topic, as described previously. Study results may also be presented by each research question, whereby study findings from one method of data collection may align with a specific study objective, whereas for others results from several research methods may be integrated. Whenever results are integrated from different methods of data collection, the source of data reported needs to be made clear for the readers, so that results can be properly interpreted.

Key Points

....

- Qualitative research generates a different type of evidence to quantitative studies, which presents different writing challenges.
- The purpose of the results section is to present study findings in a clear and compelling way in response to the research objectives.
- Writing provides another analytic tool in qualitative research and is often conducted simultaneous with further analysis to refine study findings.

- Study results need to be a logical outcome of the analytic approach described in the methods section; such coherence is an indicator of scientific rigor.
- Data reduction is an essential precursor to writing study results and can help identify the core message or story of the results.
- Focus group results are often presented in narrative form, and use quotations to illustrate issues presented. However, quotations should be used judiciously, presented ethically, and contribute to an overall argument.
- Results should be presented in a clear structure or coherent argument that identifies how individual issues contribute to the central message of the study.
- Focus group data provide an opportunity to present variation and nuances in issues, in addition to highlighting a common perspective. Presenting interaction can add additional insight to the issues reported.
- Study results can also be presented in visual formats, which can simplify the presentation of complex processes and make findings more accessible.
- Reflecting the context of study findings improves the understanding of the research issues.
- Study results need to be well grounded in data to avoid the criticism of making unsupported assertions.
- Focus group results are often presented as part of mixed methods research, where a key decision is whether to integrate or separate the findings of each method of data collection.

5

ASSESSING FOCUS
GROUP RESEARCH

HOW CAN THE quality of focus group research be assessed? This question is part of the broader issue of assessing qualitative research in general. Many scholars agree on the need for quality assessment for qualitative research, particularly with its growing use across multiple disciplines; however, the strategy for assessing quality remains an area of much debate and divergence. The traditional criteria for quality assessment of scientific research (objectivity, validity, and reliability) are often seen as inappropriate for assessing qualitative research because they are based on assumptions about research that stem from the positivist paradigm of quantitative measurement and experimental research. Some scholars have therefore proposed alternative criteria for the assessment of qualitative research that are more reflective of the interpretive paradigm that underlies qualitative approaches. However, others maintain that the concepts of validity and reliability are important quality measures, but they require a different approach when applied to qualitative research. In addition, multiple criteria for assessing qualitative research have been developed, but there remains no broad consensus on the suitability of generic criteria to assess the diverse range of approaches used in qualitative research. Discussions on appropriate and effective strategies for assessing the quality of qualitative research are therefore ongoing in academic literature.

This chapter begins by providing an overview of some of the challenges in assessing qualitative research in general, and the drawbacks of using generic criteria to assess qualitative research. The difficulties in applying the traditional criteria of validity and reliability for assessing qualitative research are explained, but this chapter focuses on the importance of these concepts for quality assessment and how each can be effectively used to assess qualitative research. The chapter concludes by outlining a framework for assessing focus group research by following stages of the research process to assess research design, data collection and interpretation, and presentation of research findings. These method-specific guidelines can be used to assess research articles using focus group discussions or to maintain rigor in the design of a focus group study.

Assessing Quality in Qualitative Research

Qualitative research is increasingly being used and published in a diverse range of disciplines. As a result, a greater variety of academic researchers, editors, reviewers, and funders are becoming exposed to qualitative research, yet many may have limited experience in qualitative research and its underlying principles. This has prompted renewed interest for guidance in assessing the quality of qualitative research, in particular the call for more formal criteria for quality assessment.

The call for assessment criteria for qualitative research has come from multiple sources. Academic researchers across a broad range of disciplines are now using qualitative research. The increase in mixed methods research and a movement toward interdisciplinary research has led to researchers in diverse disciplines becoming exposed to qualitative research. Researchers from varied disciplines request guidance on how to use and assess qualitative research. In response, a host of articles have been published in a variety of academic journals that highlight the value of qualitative research for a certain discipline and provide guidance on quality assessment. Qualitative research is also increasingly being published in biomedical journals; however, journal editors and reviewers often lack training in social science research, and fewer have specific expertise in qualitative research methods. This has promoted the need for criteria for quality assessment to guide the review process and inform publication decisions on qualitative manuscripts (Green & Thorogood, 2009; Flick, 2007). Some academic journals now provide guidelines for authors wishing to submit qualitative research, which often become the internal evaluation criteria for publication decisions. Research funding bodies also need to judge the quality and feasibility of research proposals that use qualitative methods. Leading funding bodies in the United Kingdom (e.g., Economic and Social Research Council) and the United States (e.g., National Institutes of Health, National Science Foundation) now provide documents to guide the assessment of qualitative research to foster a more transparent review process. Furthermore, much qualitative research is still conducted in the health sciences, which has experienced a major shift toward evidence-based health care, whereby health policy and practice is based on research evidence. Green and Thorogood (2009) state that if findings from qualitative research are to be included in research evidence that will inform clinical practice and healthcare decision-making, there needs to be some assessment of the quality of the evidence presented in qualitative studies. Policy and practice decisions based on low-quality research may lead to ineffective changes in health service delivery and wasted healthcare resources (Dixon-Woods, Shaw, Agarwal, & Smith, 2004). Overall, as qualitative research is increasingly being conducted and evaluated by disciplines less familiar with the principles and procedures of the approach, the need for transparent quality assessment strategies is becoming more pressing.

The traditional criteria for assessing scientific research (objectivity, validity, and reliability) are widely used across multiple disciplines. These concepts are derived from the natural sciences and are therefore most relevant to assessing quantitative and experimental research studies. The direct application of these concepts to qualitative research is problematic because of its interpretive approach, the iterative research process used, and the subjective nature of qualitative methods (discussed later). Therefore, many scholars have argued the need for different criteria to assess qualitative research from that used for quantitative studies; however, the question of how to assess qualitative research continues to be a challenge (Flick, 2007; Silverman, 2011a). In recent decades many criteria, guidelines, and checklists specifically tailored for assessing qualitative research have been proposed in academic literature or have emerged from scientific journals or research funding bodies in response to the needs described previously. Dixon-Woods et al. (2004) identified more than 100 different proposals on assessing quality in qualitative research, some of which, they state, adopt incompatible positions on certain issues.

Despite these attempts to develop criteria for quality assessment, there remains little consensus on appropriate strategies for assessing qualitative research. In part, this challenge relates to the nature of qualitative research itself, which is not a unified field but comprises a diverse range of methods, methodological approaches, and theoretical perspectives, making a criteria-based approach to assessment particularly difficult. For example, conducting in-depth interviews within the grounded theory approach may require different assessment criteria from in-depth interviews conducted within discourse analysis or within community-based participatory action research. Furthermore, assessing a study that used grounded theory is itself problematic. Not only is grounded theory difficult to implement in its original form, but the approach itself has evolved with each of its developers (Glaser and Strauss) taking the approach in different directions. Strauss developed the more structured procedural aspects of grounded theory, whereas Glaser retained the components of emergent discovery of the approach. Providing criteria to assess a grounded theory study is therefore far from straightforward. Several studies may have used the same method (e.g., interviews) or methodological approach (e.g., grounded theory), but require a different assessment strategy to acknowledge the diversity of methodological approaches used. Furthermore, developing a unified set of criteria for assessing qualitative research may have an undesirable outcome of favoring certain approaches over others, potentially leading researchers to write to the criteria to "tick the box" and maximize publication rather than reflect how validity was actually achieved in a study (Barbour, 2001).

A further challenge in developing quality criteria lies in determining how to assess the more interpretive elements of qualitative research. Some of the central tasks of qualitative research involve interpretation, such as code development and coding data, which can be difficult to describe and more challenging to assess. It remains difficult to develop indicators for readers to recognize the interpretive components of qualitative research, which can also be effectively operationalized so that different readers agree on whether these criteria have been met. The dilemma is that some of the most important qualities of qualitative research can be the hardest to assess (Dixon-Woods et al., 2004). Therefore, a concern of using criteria for quality assessment is the risk of giving less prominence to the interpretive elements because of their measurement difficulties, while giving undue prominence to the more tangible procedural tasks in qualitative research. One outcome may be that studies following appropriate procedures but with poor interpretation are considered better quality than those with less procedural detail but presenting rich and compelling interpretive detail (Dixon-Woods et al., 2004). Formalizing quality assessment through criteria may thus suppress the important interpretive components that are central to qualitative research.

Using generic criteria for assessing qualitative research therefore remains challenging, as does directly applying the traditional criteria of validity and reliability. However, the <u>concepts</u> of validity and reliability remain important for assessing qualitative research, but require a different application to embrace the interpretive paradigm and qualitative research. The following sections describe the challenges in using validity and reliability in their original form for assessing qualitative research, and then describe how each concept can be applied to qualitative research to effectively assess quality and scientific rigor.

Applying Validity and Reliability to Qualitative Research

Validity and reliability are well established measures of scientific rigor. However, they originate from quantitative research and their direct application to qualitative, interpretive research can be problematic, as indicated previously. In response, a range of alternative terms for assessing qualitative research have been proposed, such as "trustworthiness," "credibility," and "legitimacy," instead of validity and the terms "dependability," "consistency," "stability," and "representativeness" as alternative terms for reliability (Guest, MacQueen, & Namey, 2012). Although there are good arguments for using alternative terms, Morse, Barrett, Mayan, Olson, and Spiers (2002, p. 8) state that "the terms reliability and validity remain pertinent in qualitative inquiry and should be maintained," while also understanding their limitations for assessing qualitative research. Furthermore, Morse et al. (2002) argue that by creating alternative terms for these measures, qualitative research may be marginalized from mainstream science and the associated legitimacy it has. Despite their imperfect fit to qualitative research, the concepts of validity and reliability remain equally important for assessing qualitative research. Therefore, the remainder of this chapter uses the terms validity and reliability and describes how these concepts can be applied to qualitative research. Discussions of validity, reliability, and quality in qualitative research are extensive in published literature; this chapter provides only a summary of these concepts, their limitations, and how they can be applied to qualitative research. Although the strategies described next should enhance the credibility of a study, they are not sufficient to guarantee scientific rigor and quality, and cannot rectify a poorly conceived study, ineffective research instruments, or lack of critical analyses of data.

Validity

Scientific validity refers to "truth" or "accuracy" and may be described as "the extent to which an account accurately represents the social phenomenon to which it refers" (Hammersley, 1990, p. 57). The concept of validity originates from the positivist paradigm and applies most directly to quantitative research and the extent to which a study captures the true phenomenon. There are two components of validity: internal and external validity (Ritchie & Lewis, 2003). Internal validity refers to the extent to which a study measures what it intended to measure. External validity refers to the extent to which study findings are generalizable to a broader population outside the study itself. These constructs of validity are clearly based on the positivist paradigm of measurement and objectivity, and are less appropriate to qualitative research in their original form for the following reasons. The concept of validity assumes that there exists a single "truth" that can be captured through a research instrument, such as a survey. However, the underlying assumption of the interpretive paradigm is that there is not one truth but multiple perspectives on reality when examining social phenomenon. Therefore, validating the accuracy of an account is difficult to apply to qualitative research where multiple accounts of the same phenomenon are possible and it is the range of different perspectives that are valued. Internal validity is also based on the assumption that certain variables in a study, notably contextual factors, can be controlled in statistical tests to ensure that the analysis measures the specific variables of interest without any confounding factors. Such analytic approaches require standardized data collection and analytic techniques not available, or appropriate, for qualitative research. Furthermore, external validity involves the ability to generalize study findings, which typically requires drawing a random sample so that the study findings can be extrapolated to a broader population; however, qualitative research uses purposive (nonrandom) sampling aimed at seeking depth and richness of information not representativeness.

Although the concept of validity has its origins in measuring validity in quantitative research, "it is widely recognized that [validity] is an equally significant issue for qualitative research. But the questions posed are different ones and relate more to the validity of representation, understanding and interpretation" (Ritchie & Lewis, 2003, p. 273). Overall, validity has a different focus when applied to qualitative research where it is used to assess "the credibility and accuracy of process and outcomes associated with a research study" (Guest et al., 2012, p. 84). Internal validity involves assessing the credibility of a study, to examine whether the data and its interpretation are trustworthy and effectively portray the phenomenon examined. Providing transparency in the research process by describing all procedural tasks and decisions can demonstrate scientific rigor, which contributes to the trustworthiness of the data. Further strategies can be used to demonstrate the validity of interpretation of qualitative data, to show that they are valid representations of a phenomenon. In addition, the transferability of qualitative research findings is often used to describe external validity, to assess the context in which the results of qualitative research can be transferred to other settings or populations. Some approaches to demonstrate validity of qualitative data and the validity of its interpretation are summarized next.

Validity of Data

The validity of qualitative data refers to the extent to which the data effectively portray the phenomenon under investigation. Are the data trustworthy? Do they accurately represent the phenomenon, its variation, and nuance? Were data generated from an inductive process? The validity of data is clearly dependent on the rigor of the research process from which it was produced and the effective application of inductive data collection; therefore, it is necessary to demonstrate research procedures used to enable validity to be assessed. This requires researchers to clearly document the research process so that others can judge the credibility of the research and the trustworthiness of the data. Demonstrating credibility and showing transparency are key strategies that contribute to assessing the validity of qualitative data, as described next.

Credibility (Lincoln & Guba, 1985) refers to the trustworthiness of the study to generate valid data that accurately represent the phenomenon studied. Credibility refers to the "confidence in the truth of the findings, including an accurate understanding of the context" (Ulin, Robinson, & Tolley, 2005, p. 25). Assessing whether data collected effectively reflect the views of study participants is central to assessing qualitative research. The credibility of the study is directly related to the research process, the methodological procedures and decisions, and the steps taken to ensure scientific rigor. Therefore, validity can be enhanced during all stages of the research process from developing an appropriate research design, selecting research methods, following inductive data collection, and using effective strategies to analyze and interpret data. At each of these stages of the research process scientific rigor can be enhanced, such as adequate training of moderators on rapport development and probing; pilot-testing discussion questions; following inductive data collection (described later); using accepted procedures for data analysis to ensure interpretations are evidence based; and implementing ethical procedures. Scientific rigor through all stages of the research process is critical for data validity. Therefore, validity is not only assessed at the completion of a study but addressed during each task in the research process. Providing transparency in reporting the research process (see discussion below) can demonstrate that the research is robust and that procedural validity was enhanced throughout the study. For focus group research, the elements of effective study design and implementation have been described in previous chapters of this book. Figure 5.1 details specific questions that can be asked of a focus group study to assess its credibility.

Inductive data collection, using open questions and probing participants, inherently facilitates valid responses from participants, particularly compared with structured quantitative data collection. Guest et al. (2012) state that the open-ended nature of interview questions and inductive probing used in qualitative research allow researchers to gain more precise responses from participants than closed category questions on a survey instrument. For example, a participant's response to a survey question may not be offered as one of the closed category options in quantitative research, particularly when there is no "other" category. This leaves the participants or the interviewer to assign a response category, which may not be entirely valid. This problem is avoided in qualitative research where participants can provide open and elaborate responses in their own words without the constraint of researchers' categories, which may more accurately capture their views and provide greater depth and nuance, thereby improving data validity and overall quality. In addition, the interviewer has the flexibility to probe a participant for clarity or rephrase a question if it seems unclear to a participant. Therefore, the interactive and inductive processes of qualitative interviewing inherently contribute to data validity.

Transparency involves clearly reporting the research process to provide an "audit trail" of procedures and decisions from which others can assess the validity of the study and the data generated. An audit trail lays bare the rationale for the study design, the process of data generation, and the analytic procedures used. It not only provides procedural information on what was done and who was involved, but also the reasoning for choices made during the research process. In addition, an audit trail can "show the conceptual process by which meaning or interpretation has been attributed or theory developed" (Ritchie & Lewis, 2003, p. 276). Therefore, an effective audit trail highlights the analytic steps that led to assertions made in the findings, so that there are no seemingly unsupported leaps of logic in the final results presented. Providing transparency in the research process is particularly important in qualitative research given the diversity of approaches used and the iterative process of data collection. This diversity means that studies using similar research methods may have applied a different field approach, which underscores the need for each study to clearly document their process, procedures, and rationale. Although such documentation does not guarantee validity, it does provide important information for readers to make an informed assessment of the scientific rigor of the study, and thereby the credibility of the study findings and interpretations. The importance of transparency is not only for external quality assessment, but can also encourage researchers to be more systematic and deliberate in their approach and provide clear rationale for the methodological decisions, thereby also increasing research quality throughout the study (Guest et al., 2012).

Validity of Interpretation

Much qualitative research is based on understanding meaning and interpretation of data. Therefore, demonstrating the validity of these interpretations is critical to the trustworthiness of qualitative research findings. How valid are researchers' understandings and interpretation of the data collected? How can researchers' manage subjective interpretation of data? How can validity of concepts and explanations be demonstrated? These are critical questions in assessing the validity of interpretation in qualitative research. Several strategies are commonly used to demonstrate the validity of researcher's interpretations of qualitative data, as described next.

Respondent validation (also called "member checking") involves presenting a summary of the study findings to a selection of study participants, other members of the study population, or key informants familiar with the culture or context of the research. These informants are asked to respond to the research findings, often confirming or clarifying results presented, and verifying their accuracy within the study population. This strategy provides some external validation that study results and their interpretation are valid and recognizable by members of the study community themselves. It provides an important safeguard against interpretation bias. When this strategy is used it is typically included in the methods section of a research article, highlighting the nature of the respondents providing comment and whether any discrepancies in interpretation were identified.

Although respondent validation has some appeal, it presents numerous challenges. Data are collected from individual participants, yet respondent validation involves verifying the collective study results that comprise a synthesis of multiple experiences and perspectives. Some have questioned the effectiveness of this approach. Can study participants effectively verify analytic outcomes of a study, which result from cross-case comparison and detailed immersion in data? Will study participants understand the collective results of academic research? Some scholars (Morse et al., 2002; Barbour, 2001; Mays & Pope, 2000) caution that respondent validation may be problematic because an individual's response may not be visible in aggregated research results. This becomes particularly challenging when study results are more conceptual or present explanatory frameworks, such as in grounded theory, because concepts and processes become more abstract than the individual experiences from which they are generated and may therefore be difficult to recognize by the study community. In contrast, Guest et al. (2012) believe that even though an individual's response is not explicitly visible, participants would be able to recognize some of the issues that their contribution helped to create. A related challenge in using this method of validation is that it assumes that a single reality is being verified; however, multiple experiences were captured in the data. This may cause participants to disagree with the experiences or viewpoints presented in the results that they are unfamiliar with or that differ from their own perspectives. This does not mean that these results are incorrect, but reflects that multiple perspectives exist. Thus, participants may validate their own perspective but not that of others as presented in study results. Furthermore, respondent validation may not be logistically feasible when it is not possible to return to the study population, such as for in international research or when resources are limited.

Peer review involves assessing validity by asking researchers outside the research team to examine study data and the interpretations derived. This provides an assessment of "external validity." Peers are instructed to assess the logic and consistency of the analysis to identify potential interpretation bias (Guest et al., 2012). Peer review provides assessment of the researchers' interpretations and whether these are well-grounded in the data itself, thereby keeping researchers' subjectivity in check. A similar strategy can be conducted within the study team, whereby several team members analyze the same section of data independently to assess the consistency with which they are able to generate similar interpretations of the data.

Negative and deviant case analyses are strategies for increasing analytic rigor to minimize researcher's interpretation bias. Qualitative research is commonly criticized for using data selectively (or "cherry-picking") to support an argument proposed by the researcher. Negative and deviant case analyses are analytic tasks that challenge researchers to be critically self-reflective in interpreting data by challenging their interpretations. Negative case analysis involves actively seeking data that may contradict themes identified or an explanation proposed, and highlighting or explaining these negative cases. Contradictory data can be challenging to manage but explicitly seeking and incorporating these data into the study results indicates that data interpretations are indeed reflective of complex qualitative analysis rather than being used selectively to support a particular perspective. Similarly, deviant case analysis involves identifying outliers that do not fit an emerging interpretation of the data. These outliers are then examined explicitly, whereby researchers may adjust their interpretations to incorporate outliers or understand why these cases are different. These strategies may be reported in the data analysis section of a research article to demonstrate how the interpretations presented "fit" the study data.

Delimiting interpretations to make explicit the context in which they are valid is a simple strategy to increase the validity of interpretations presented. Not all study findings are relevant to the entire study population. Some explanations apply to a defined subset of participants (e.g., young males only), whereas others are valid only under certain conditions or circumstances (e.g., only participants who use public transport explained difficulties in accessing facilities). Delineating the boundaries, or scope, of an explanation provides specificity on when an explanation is valid and the conditions under which this interpretation holds true, thereby increasing the validity of interpretation.

Analytic induction is a process of analyzing qualitative data involving iterative interpretation to ensure that explanations "fit" the data. Analytic induction (Silverman, 2011a; Flick, 2009; Fielding, 1988) involves developing a provisional explanation of phenomenon based on initial analyses, then examining data case by case to assess whether the explanation fits each case. As each case is examined the explanation is adjusted to incorporate nuances of specific cases, so that the explanation evolves from the analytic process. When a case does not fit, the explanation is refined and this process continues until all data can be accounted for with the final explanation. Analytic induction involves constant comparison of cases; examination of negative cases; and incorporation of outliers (described above). The use of analytic induction strengthens study findings by demonstrating that they originate from data itself and not researchers' subjective interpretation. Although the details of each iteration are not reported in a research article, the use of analytic induction and any major adjustments to an explanation may be noted in a description of data analysis and theory building.

Triangulation refers to "combining multiple theories, methods, observers and empirical materials, to produce a more accurate, comprehensive and objective representation of the object of study" (Silverman, 2011a, p. 369). It is a common strategy for validating research findings that is based on the premise that when findings from multiple independent sources converge it provides confidence that the findings are trustworthy and valid.

Triangulation may contribute to validity in two ways: by confirmation of the study findings or by providing completeness of the findings. Denzin (1989) suggests four ways to use triangulation as confirmation of study findings in qualitative research by triangulating: (1) between research approaches (e.g., quantitative and qualitative); (2) between methods (e.g., interviews and group discussions); (3) between researchers (e.g., using multiple interviewers or analysts); and (4) theory triangulation, whereby data are viewed through different theoretical lenses. Using multiple methods and multiple approaches are perhaps the most common applications of triangulation in qualitative research, in addition to comparing coding from independent analysts to confirm similar understanding and interpretation of data between researchers. A further strategy involves comparing study findings with themes, concepts, and interpretations provided in extant literature among similar study populations.

Triangulation may also be used to improve the completeness of qualitative study findings. Triangulation may be used as a means to increase understanding of phenomenon by examining it from different perspectives, thereby exploiting the variation sought in qualitative research. This use of triangulation does not validate or confirm findings but "is best understood as a strategy that adds rigor, breadth, complexity, richness and depth to any enquiry" (Denzin & Lincoln, 2000, p. 5). This approach adds rigor to the research by exploring phenomenon from multiple perspectives, examining contradictions and inconsistencies that exist in qualitative data to provide a fuller understanding of the issues.

Using triangulation to confirm study findings has ready appeal, but it can be difficult to conduct effectively. Data from different methods come in very different forms (e.g., observations vs. group discussions vs. survey data) that may not be directly comparable. Furthermore, the generation of similar findings from different methods of data collection provides some confirmation of those findings, but the absence of corroboration does not suggest lack of validity in qualitative research, because different methods produce different views of the phenomenon under study (Barbour, 2001). There is also some debate among qualitative researchers on the value of triangulation for confirming study findings, because it assumes there is a single objective truth that can be validated. However, "in cultural research, which focuses on social reality, the object of knowledge *is* different from different perspectives. And the different points of view cannot be merged, into a single, 'true' and 'certain' representation of the object" (Moisander & Valtonen, 2006, p. 45). Hammersley (1992) argues that one cannot know for certain that accounts given in social research are true because there is no independent and reliable access to "reality," therefore all accounts can be true even when divergent, because they represent different perspectives on reality. It is often the goal of qualitative research to seek out variant views and diverse experiences, therefore assessing validity by convergence (through triangulation) seems contradictory to the purpose of qualitative research. Nevertheless, some applications of triangulation can validate study findings in qualitative research, so triangulation should not be dismissed but applied with awareness of its limitations for validating social research.

External Validity

External validity typically refers to the ability to generalize study findings to a broader population. It is an important criterion for validity in quantitative research. Generalizability is based on the expectation of a sufficiently large sample whereby participants are randomly selected and standardized data collection is used. As such, generalizability is difficult to apply to qualitative research, which focuses on a small number of participants selected non-randomly and data are collected using responsive (non-standardized) interviewing, because the goal is to seek information richness not representation. Some scholars state that generalizability is not applicable to qualitative research because it is based purely on description and focuses on select cases. Others state that generalization is a relevant and achievable task in qualitative research, albeit conducted in a different way than in quantitative studies. For example, Padgett (2012, p. 206) states that "[qualitative] findings can have transferability and resonance without being 'generalizable' in a statistical sense based on how the sample was selected," and Mason (1996, p. 6) states that "qualitative research should produce explanations which are generalizable in some way, or have wider resonance." Given that the concept of generalizability may be difficult to apply to qualitative research, Lincoln and Guba (1985) suggest the term "transferability of study findings" as more appropriate for qualitative research.

In qualitative research, generalization is approached differently than in quantitative research. Ritchie and Lewis (2003) describe three forms of generalizability for qualitative research: (1) representational generalizability, (2) inferential generalizability, and (3) theoretical generalizability. Representational generalizability refers to the extent to which study findings can be inferred to the parent population from which they were sampled; however, the basis for such representation is different in qualitative research. In qualitative research "it is not the prevalence of particular views or experiences... about which wider inferences can be drawn. Rather, it is the content or 'map' of the range of views, experiences, outcomes or other phenomena under study and the factors and circumstances that shape and influence them, that can be inferred to the research population... It is at the level of categories, concepts and explanation that generalization can take place" (Ritchie & Lewis, 2003, p. 269). Achieving representational generalizability draws on issues of validity of the research process, including the degree to which the sample captures diversity within the parent population and the accuracy with which phenomenon have been identified and interpreted (as described in previous sections). For example, using recruitment strategies for maximum variation (e.g., purposive and theoretical sampling) captures diversity in the context and conditions of the issues examined, thereby capturing the heterogeneity within the parent population that enables inferences to become applicable. This aspect of generalizability reflects the principle of statistical inference but without using probability criteria. It refers more to achieving inclusivity and diversity in the dimensions and properties of the issues examined (Silverman, 2011a). The validity and scientific rigor of a study therefore has a critical influence on achieving representational generalizability.

Inferential generalizability refers to the relevance of the study findings to other contexts and populations beyond the study setting itself. For example, as the extent to which findings from a study on injecting drug users in New York City can be applied to injecting drug users in other large US cities. The core distinction from representational generalizability is that findings are not so much being assessed as "representing" the parent population, although this is implicit, but being applied (or "inferred") to a new context or population. Inferential generalizability is achieved in qualitative research by generating broader level concepts, processes, explanations, or theoretical frameworks that have relevance outside the specific context from which they were derived. For example, such general concepts as "fear," "stigma," "peer pressure," or "bullying" are transferable to other contexts, but the specific examples from which these concepts were derived remain context- or case-specific. Therefore, "[inferential] generalization in qualitative research is the gradual transfer of findings from case studies and their context to more general and abstract relations, for example a typology" (Flick, 2009, p. 408). This involves reducing the contextual relevance of the study findings by developing broader conceptual results that can be transferred to other settings. Flick (2009, p. 407) states that "this attachment to contexts often allows qualitative research a specific expressiveness. However, when attempts are made at generalizing the findings, this context link has to be given up in order to find out whether the findings are valid independently of and outside specific contexts." Some approaches to qualitative research, such as grounded theory, are more suited to generating conceptual results from individual narrative experiences. It is important to document the analytic process by which broader concepts were derived to demonstrate the internal validity of those concepts being transferred. The effectiveness of inferential generalizability undoubtedly also depends on external factors, such as the degree of congruence between the study context and the context to which findings are being inferred. Providing as much contextual detail as possible on the study itself allows others to determine the appropriateness of inferring findings to other contexts.

Finally, theoretical generalizability refers to the use of study results to develop empirical theory, by the development of new theory or the contribution of new concepts to existing theory. In this sense the theory developed is context-free and thus generalizable in the universal sense as a contribution to scientific inquiry. However generalization is used in qualitative research, the type of generalization and the basis for its relevance needs to be made clear so that appropriate claims of generalizability can be made.

Reliability

Reliability refers to the replicability of a study, whereby if the study was repeated using the same methods and approach it could produce the same results. Reliability responds to the question of "whether or not some future researchers could repeat the research project and come up with the same results, interpretations and claims" (Silverman, 2011a, p. 360). It is an objective measure of consistency, which essentially demonstrates that the study findings are independent of any accidental circumstance of their production, and are therefore free of subjectivity or bias (Kirk & Miller, 1986). Reliability originates from the natural sciences and is most appropriate to more standardized quantitative research and experimental design, whereby taking repeated measures that show consistent results demonstrates the reliability of those readings.

The ideal of objective replicability is often seen as unobtainable in qualitative research because of the subjective nature of social research and the iterative research process used. Qualitative research is often conducted to understand complex social phenomenon, to explore contextual influences on social behavior, and to seek diversity in participants' experiences and characteristics. To do this it requires an iterative process of discovery that is responsive and dynamic so that researchers can follow leads as the research process unfolds. This approach is unlikely to be repeated exactly; therefore, the goal of objective replication may be naive and unachievable in qualitative research (Lincoln & Guba, 1985). Even when using semi-structured research instruments, which often ask the same open questions in the same order, an interviewer often uses a great deal of responsive probing thereby taking each interview in potentially very different directions depending on the participant's experiences (Guest et al., 2012). Therefore, even though structure may exist in qualitative research instruments, inductive probing means that responses may not be replicable, but this is not to say that these responses are not reliable.

Replicability may also be challenging because of the interpretive nature of qualitative research. Interpretation is a central component of qualitative research, but it introduces subjective influences to the research process, which challenge the goal of replicability. These concerns mean that the goal of objective replicability, which is implicit in reliability, is not appropriate to qualitative research. However, this does not mean that the concept of reliability should be abandoned altogether for qualitative studies, but rather discussed in terms that have greater resonance with the principles and procedures of qualitative research. As a result of these issues alternative terms have been proposed for assessing reliability in qualitative research, for example "confirmability" (Ritchie & Lewis, 2003); "consistency" (Hammersley, 1990); "trustworthiness" (Glaser & Strauss, 1967); "dependability" (Lincoln & Guba, 1985); and "transparency" (Silverman, 2011a). These terms highlight central characteristics of reliability but do not focus on objective replicability.

Reliability is often seen as less important than validity in qualitative research because replication, which is at the heart of reliability, is not a goal of qualitative research. In applying reliability to qualitative research, it is important to understand the elements of qualitative research that can be consistent and confirmed, and that could reoccur with some certainty. Ritchie and Lewis (2003, p. 271) state that "it is the collective nature of the phenomena that have been generated by the study participants and the meanings that they have attached to them that would be expected to repeat." Therefore, replicability may be sought in the core concepts identified in qualitative data and the consistency in understanding the meanings that participants attach to these concepts; "thus the reliability of the findings depends on the likely recurrence of the original data and the way they are interpreted" (Ritchie & Lewis, 2003, p. 271). Reliability rests in part on rigorous application of qualitative research procedures to identify inductive constructs and their interpretation, and on transparency and documentation of these procedures. In this way reliability also enhances the validity of a study. Reliability becomes particularly relevant to qualitative research when comparison is sought, for example between groups or locations, requiring some consistency in study procedures. Providing structure in research procedures facilitates reliability and comparison. Guest et al. (2012, p. 88) highlight that "instruments, questions and processes with more structure enable a more meaningful comparative analysis. With no structure one cannot make claims that any differences observed are due to actual differences between groups, since all or most of the variability could just as easily be due to differences in the way questions were asked." Structure may be achieved by using systematic procedures in data collection and analysis; however, these should not compromise the inductive discovery that is characteristic of qualitative inquiry. Strategies for building structure in qualitative research to enhance comparability and reliability have been well documented and are summarized next.

Transparency of research procedures is as important for reliability as it is for validity (as described previously). Detailed documentation of the scientific procedures used in data collection and analysis are critical for the replicability of a study, and demonstrate that data support the claims made in the study findings. Furthermore, Silverman (2011a) indicates the importance of "theoretical transparency" for assessing reliability, whereby researchers make explicit the theoretical stance from which interpretation was conducted, and show how this led to the particular interpretations of data that were presented and excluded other interpretations, thereby guiding the reader on the theoretical framework within which the study could be reliably replicated. It is therefore incumbent on researchers to provide sufficient detail and transparency on the research process, procedures, and the theoretical stance of the study to assess its reliability (Kirk & Miller, 1986).

Reflexivity involves researchers indicating subjective characteristics or circumstances that may have influenced data collection or interpretation. Reflexivity is an important element of reliability because it can indicate whether there were certain characteristics of the researcher (e.g., ethnicity, experience, perspectives, or language ability) that may have influenced the nature of data collected. Similarly, specific circumstances may be unique to a study, for example a study on people's perceptions of disaster relief immediately after experiencing an earthquake, drought, or other natural disaster. These characteristics and circumstances may be unique to a particular study and not replicable in future studies. Therefore, including reflexivity in a research report is important for its influence on the replicability of a study. Reflexivity therefore extends the transparency of the research process and contributes to assessing reliability.

Using systematic procedures provides consistency in the research process, which supports reliability. The systematic procedures that may be used for focus group discussions are described more fully in Chapter 2. For example, using a semistructured discussion guide ensures participants are asked the same set of open questions, while still allowing the moderator to explore issues raised in the discussion. Field-testing the discussion guide provides a check on whether participants consistently understand the questions in the same way. Training moderators on the intent of each question on the discussion guide facilitates relevant and consistent probing, because "without a sense of purpose, inductive probing lacks both direction and relevance" (Guest et al., 2012, p. 86). Monitoring data as they are collected improves consistency and overall data quality, as it provides an opportunity to review transcripts or debrief with moderators to refocus questioning strategies when needed. Recording interviews, verbatim transcription, and accurate translation of data have become the norm in many qualitative studies. These procedures ensure that data represent participants' own words and intents as concretely as possible and therefore generate more accurate data. Using a transcription protocol adds consistency and systematic rigor, as does checking transcripts for accuracy and completeness (Hennink, 2007, 2008). Translating data adds complexity to data reliability, but training translators on developing verbatim translated transcripts that retain the intent of the speaker contributes to consistency. Use of data analysis software can also improve systematic data analysis. These procedures provide structure and reliability checking at important stages during the process of generating focus group data.

Verbatim quotations connect a reader directly to the words of a study participant, and provide a direct link between the issues raised by participants and their interpretation by researchers. Quotations therefore provide a powerful contribution to reliability in qualitative research, because "quotes lay bare the emergent themes for all to see" (Guest et al., 2012, p. 95). They enable issues to be verified in the direct words of a participant, rather than relying only on researchers' interpretation of the issues (Seale, 1999), thereby improving transparency and reliability. However, quotations should always be part of a narrative; without this it can have a detrimental effect on reliability because readers are then open to draw their own interpretations based on select quotations and without having had the benefit of analyzing the whole data set (see Chapter 4 on presenting quotations from focus group research).

Inter-coder reliability is perhaps the most commonly described measure of reliability in qualitative research (Guest et al., 2012; Silverman, 2011a; Barbour, 2001). Inter-coder reliability typically involves two analysts who independently code the same transcripts with an identical set of codes and then compare the consistency of their coding. It provides a strong reliability check to assess whether different researchers interpret qualitative data in the same way by identifying the same core concepts and then code data in a consistent way, thus minimizing subjective interpretation. Developing a codebook that lists all codes and a detailed description of their application adds consistency between coders. There are three common methods to assess inter-coder agreement (Guest et al., 2012; Silverman, 2011a).

Subjective assessment involves coders simply discussing the double-coded text to identify discrepancies in interpretation of data and application of codes, and then revising the codebook or coding strategies if needed. No metrics are generated with this method.

Percent agreement calculates simple percentage agreement based on the tally of agreements over the total number of comparisons. Some qualitative data analysis software has this function and generates tables of agreement by codes or coders, and calculates an overall percentage agreement. This method is useful for identifying problematic codes, coders, or coding strategies used. An overall percentage agreement of 80% or higher is considered good agreement.

Cohen's kappa calculates the level of agreement taking into account chance agreement and is therefore considered more accurate. A kappa score of 0.8 or greater is considered high, but often difficult to achieve. Cohen's kappa is not effective for small samples and an overreliance on a single statistical score can detract from focusing on the causes of coding discrepancies that influence reliability.

With all methods of intercoder reliability an important component is identifying the causes of coding discrepancies, such as problems with codes, different interpretation of data, or variations in coding styles, and then rectifying these issues. Typically codes that have less than 80% simple agreement or a kappa score of below 0.8 are discussed and revised to improve consistency. Although producing a quantitative measure of intercoder agreement has its place there are also limitations. For example, even a slight difference in the size of a coded text segment coded is considered inconsistent agreement reducing the level of agreement generated. Therefore, simple subjective assessment often is sufficient and retains the focus on discussing discrepancies to increase consistency.

Assessing Focus Group Research

The applications of validity and reliability discussed previously are relevant for assessing focus group research. The strategies described in this chapter can be used to determine the overall credibility of a focus group study to produce valid data and to assess the trustworthiness of a researcher's interpretations of data. Following the procedural guidance given throughout this book will assist in making effective methodological decisions to improve the quality and rigor of a focus group study and contribute to valid and reliable study outcomes.

In assessing focus group research it can be helpful to adopt a process approach to examine whether aspects of validity and reliability are addressed at different stages of the research process. Figure 5.1 integrates relevant procedural advice on conducting focus group research (given in this book) with indicators of validity and reliability (discussed in this chapter) and presents questions that can be asked at different stages of the research process

STUDY PURPOSE	
Study Purpose	Is the study purpose clearly stated?
	Does the article title effectively capture the study purpose?
	Are focus group discussions the most effective method for the study purpose?
	Is the significance of the study clearly articulated?
Research Question	Is the research question clear and focused?
	Is the research question suitable for qualitative research?
	Are focus group discussions suitable to answer the research question?
RESEARCH DESIGN	
Theoretical Framework	Is the study embedded in a theoretical framework?
Study Design	Is the study design clearly identified?
	Does the study design operationalize the theoretical framework?
	Are focus group discussions appropriate for the study design?
	Is the use of focus group discussions clearly justified?
	Is the role of focus group discussions clear in a mixed methods study design?
DATA COLLECTION	
Context	Is the study context sufficiently described?
	Is the selection of study sites described?
Field Team	Is it clear who collected the data and their characteristics?
	Are the moderator(s) characteristics described?
	Was there a note-taker present at the focus groups?
	Is training of the field team described?
Participants	Is the study population defined?
	Was the study population segmented in any way?
	Are the types of study participants recruited appropriate for the study purpose?
	Do they appear to be the most 'information rich' sources on the topic?

Figure 5.1. Assessing focus group research.

Recruitment	Are the inclusion/exclusion criteria made clear?
	Is participant selection theoretically justified?
	Is the process of participant recruitment described in detail?
	Are recruitment strategies relevant to the study population?
	Was participant recruitment iterative?
Group Size, Composition & Number	Is the size of focus groups appropriate? Are particularly small/large groups justified?
	Is group composition homogeneous? How was this achieved?
	Is the level of acquaintance between participants indicated (e.g. strangers or acquaintances)?
	Is the number of focus groups stated and justified?
Data Collection	When were data collected?
	Is there evidence of iterative data collection?
	How was group interaction encouraged?
	Is there evidence of responsive probing?
	How was information saturation achieved/ determined?
	Were focus groups held in a suitable location?
	Is the context of data collection reflected?
	Is an audit trail of data collection and analysis evident?
Research Instrument	Was a discussion guide used?
	Does the discussion guide operationalize the study objectives?
	Are the topics or questions asked described? Are they suitable for a group discussion?
	Are questions open and designed to promote discussion?
	Are questions culturally appropriate for the study population?
	Is the number of questions appropriate?
	Was the discussion guide piloted?
	Was it translated and checked for accuracy?

Figure 5.1. (Continued)

Reflexivity	Is there evidence of reflexivity during the research process?
	Do researchers reflect whether characteristics of the moderator, group location or contextual issues may have influenced data collection?
Ethics	Was ethical approval received?
	Are ethical issues adequately described?
	How was the research explained to participants?
	How was informed consent achieved?
	How were anonymity and confidentiality of participants protected?
	How were risks to participants minimized?
DATA	
Data Recording	How were data recorded?
	Were group discussions transcribed verbatim and/or translated?
	How were transcriptions/ translations checked for accuracy?
Data	Is there evidence of 'thick' data with depth, breadth, context and nuance?
	Does the data retain the 'voices' of the participants?
Analysis	Is the analytic approach stated and appropriate?
	Were data analyzed systematically?
	Is the process of data analysis clearly described, allowing the reader to see how analysis was conducted and results were derived?
	Is there adequate description of how codes and concepts were derived from the data?
	How was code development and coding of data validated?
	Is it clear whether data analysis was inductive?
	How were study findings validated?
	How was interpretation bias managed?
	Was a theoretical framework used to guide data analysis?
	Are negative cases discussed and explained?

Figure 5.1. (Continued)

Limitations	Are limitations of the data, method or study described?
STUDY RESULTS	
Clear & Coherent	Are the study results described clearly? Do the study results reflect the application of the analytic approach stated? Is there logical coherence between the methods, results and study conclusions? Do results respond effectively to study purpose and research question? Is it clear how data collection and analysis arrived at the findings presented?
Structure	Is there a clear and logical structure, argument or central message conveyed? Is there a clear distinction between presentation of data and their interpretation? Are results from different methods presented effectively? Is the data source of results indicated (if different types of data are used)?
New Knowledge	Did new or unanticipated issues emerge from data? Is sufficient context of findings presented to determine their transferability? Is the significance of the results made clear?
Variation	Are a range of issues reported? Are diverse views described? Were effective comparisons made and reported? Was group interaction evident in the study results?
Depth & Focus	Are issues described in depth and detail? Are specific examples provided? Are nuances of issues described? Do results focus on responding to the research question?

Figure 5.1. (Continued)

Context	Is the context of each issue described?
	Do the recommendations consider the broader socio-cultural or political context?
	Can participants 'voices' be distinguished from their interpretation by researchers?
	Are study findings placed in the context of the research literature on the topic?
Presentation	Are results presented appropriately within the interpretive paradigm?
	Are diagrams or visual displays of results effective?
	Are results presented ethically?
	Are quotations used effectively to support study findings?
	Are participants' identities protected in reporting of quotations?
Validity	Have effective strategies been used to validate data and its interpretation?
	Are study findings effectively grounded in the data?
	Are assertions made supported by the data?
	Is there sufficient evidence presented to validate findings?
DISCUSSION & CONCLUSION	
Appropriate	Are study implications clearly articulated?
	Are the implications adequately supported by study data?
	Is the transferability of results appropriately discussed?
	Are conclusions based on the research evidence?
	Is further research suggested?

Figure 5.1. (Continued)

to assess the quality and rigor of focus group research. This framework operationalizes the concepts of quality assessment into practical questions that can be used to judge the quality of focus group research. The framework may be used when writing or reviewing focus group research. The questions are presented as a guide rather than a mandate for assessing focus group research. Finally, given the word limits of journal articles not all procedural details and justifications can be included in a research article; therefore, a balance between ideal content and practical realities also needs to be considered when evaluating focus group research.

Key Points

....

- Applying traditional quality assessment criteria (objectivity, validity, and reliability) to qualitative research can be problematic because of the interpretive approach, iterative research process, and subjectivity of qualitative research.
- Alternative strategies, checklists, criteria, and terminology for assessing qualitative research have been proposed, but there remains no agreement on appropriate assessment of qualitative research.
- The concepts of validity and reliability remain important for qualitative research, but they require a different application to effectively assess qualitative inquiry.
- Assessing validity of data and its interpretation is important in qualitative research. Rather than measuring validity, it is the validity of representation, understanding, and interpretation that is assessed in qualitative research.
- Strategies for assessing data validity include credibility of the research process and transparency in documenting research procedures.
- Strategies for assessing data interpretation include respondent validation, peer review, negative and deviant case analysis, delimiting interpretations, analytic induction, triangulation, and transferability.
- Assessing reliability in qualitative research focuses on identifying whether there is recurrence of core concepts and consistent meaning of these concepts in data.
- Strategies for assessing reliability in qualitative research include using structure and systematic procedures to identify core concepts (e.g., training data collectors, recording data, verbatim transcription, pilot testing instruments, inter-coder reliability, reporting verbatim quotations, and using reflexivity).
- Focus group research may be assessed using a process approach to identify how validity and reliability were addressed at different stages of the research process (see Figure 5.1).

6

FURTHER READING AND RESOURCES

Introduction to Focus Group Discussions

Barbour, R. (2007). *Doing focus groups.* The SAGE Qualitative Research Kit. London: Sage Publications.

Bloor, M., Frankland, J., Thomas, M., & Robson, K. (2001). *Focus groups in social research.*London: Sage Publications.

Fox, F., Morris, M., & Rumsey, N. (2007). Doing synchronous online focus groups with young people: Methodological reflections. *Qualitative Health Research,* 17(4), 539–547.

Hennink, M. (2007). *International focus group research: A handbook for the health and social sciences.* Cambridge: Cambridge University Press.

Kitzinger, J., & Barbour, R. (1999). Introduction: The challenge and promise of focus groups. In R. Barbour & J. Kitzinger (Eds.), *Developing focus group research: Politics, theory and practice* (pp. 1–20). London: Sage Publications.

Krueger, R., & Casey, M. (2009). *Focus groups: A practical guide for applied research* (4th ed.). Thousand Oaks, CA: Sage Publications.

Liamputtong, P. (2011). *Focus group methodology.* London: Sage Publications.

Planning, Conducting, and Analyzing Focus Group Research

Barbour, R. (2007). *Doing focus groups.* The SAGE Qualitative Research Kit. London: Sage Publications.

Bernard, H., & Ryan, G. (2010). *Analyzing qualitative data: Systematic approaches.* Thousand Oaks, CA: Sage Publications.

Charmaz, K. (2006). *Constructing grounded theory: A practical guide through qualitative analysis.* London: Sage Publications.

Colucci, E. (2007). Focus groups can be fun: The use of activity oriented questions in focus group discussions. *Qualitative Health Research*, 17(10), 1422–1433.

Denzin, N., & Lincoln, Y. (Eds.). (2008). *Collecting and interpreting qualitative materials* (3rd ed.). Thousand Oaks, CA: Sage Publications.

Dickson-Swift, V., James, E., Kippen, S., & Liamputtong, P. (2008). Risks to researchers in qualitative research on sensitive topics: Issues and strategies. *Qualitative Health Research*, 18(1), 133–144.

Elliott, J. (2005). *Using narrative in social research: Qualitative and quantitative approaches.* London: Sage Publications.

Esposito, N. (2001). From meaning to meaning: The influence of translation techniques on non-English focus group research. *Qualitative Health Research*, 11(4), 568–579.

Glaser, B., & Strauss, A. (1967). *The discovery of grounded theory: Strategies for qualitative research.* New York: Aldine de Gruyter.

Grbich, C. (2007). *Qualitative data analysis: An introduction.* London: Sage Publications.

Guest, G., MacQueen, K., & Namey, E. (2012). *Applied thematic analysis.* Thousand Oaks, CA: Sage.

Guest, G., Bunce, A., & Johnson, L. (2006). How many interviews are enough? An experiment with data saturation and variability. *Field Methods*, 18, 59–82.

Hennink, M. (2007). *International focus group research: A handbook for the health and social sciences.* Cambridge: Cambridge University Press.

Hennink, M. (2008). Language and communication in cross-cultural research. In P. Liamputtong (Ed.), *Doing cross-cultural research: Ethical and methodological considerations.* Springer.

Hennink, M., Hutter, I., & Bailey, A. (2011). *Qualitative research methods.* London: Sage Publications.

Krippendorf, K. (2004). *Content analysis: An introduction to its methodology* (2nd ed.). Thousand Oaks, CA: Sage.

Krueger, R., & Casey, M. (2009). *Focus groups: A practical guide for applied research* (4th ed.). Thousand Oaks, CA: Sage Publications.

MacDougall, C., & Fudge, E. (2001). Planning and recruiting the sample for focus groups and in-depth interviews. *Qualitative Health Research*, 11(1), 117–126.

Maynard-Tucker, G. (2000). Conducting focus groups in developing countries: Skill training for local bilingual facilitators. *Qualitative Health Research*, 10, 396–410.

Morse, J. (2000). Editorial: Determining sample size. *Qualitative Health Research*, 10(1), 3–5.

O'Donnell, A., Lutfey, K., Marceau, L., & McKinlay, J. (2007). Using focus groups to improve validity of cross-national survey research: A study of physician decision making. *Qualitative Health Research*, 17(17), 971–981.

Phillips, N., & Hardy, C. (2002). *Discourse analysis: Investigating processes of social construction.* Qualitative Research Methods Series, Vol. 50. Thousand Oaks, CA: Sage Publications.

Rapley, T. (2007). *Doing conversation, discourse and document analysis. The SAGE Qualitative Research Kit.* London: Sage Publications.

Silverman, D. (2011a). *Interpreting qualitative data* (4th ed.). London: Sage Publications.

Strauss, A., & Corbin, J. (1998). *Basics of qualitative research: Techniques and procedures for developing grounded theory* (2nd ed.). Thousand Oaks, CA: Sage Publications.

Weber, R. (1990). *Basic content analysis* (2nd ed.). Newbury Park, CA: Sage.

Wilkinson, S. (2011). Analysing focus group data. In D. Silverman (Ed.), *Qualitative research* (3rd ed., pp. 168–186). London: Sage

Writing Qualitative Research

Belgrave, L., Zablotsky, D., & Guadagno, M. (2002). How do we talk to each other? Writing qualitative research for quantitative readers. *Qualitative Health Research*, 12(10), 1427–1439.

Duggleby, W. (2005). What about focus group interaction data? *Qualitative Health Research*, 15(6), 832–840.

Guest, G., MacQueen, K., & Namey, E. (2012). Writing up thematic analyses. In Applied thematic analysis (pp. 241–272). Thousand Oaks, CA: Sage.

Hennink, M., Hutter, I., & Bailey, A. (2011). Writing qualitative research. In *Qualitative research methods* (Chapter 11). (pp. 268–293). London: Sage Publications.

Mason, J. (2002). Making convincing arguments with qualitative data. In *Qualitative researching* (2nd ed., pp. 173–204). London: Sage Publications.

Morgan, D. (2010). Reconsidering the role of interaction in analysing and reporting focus groups. *Qualitative Health Research*, 20(5), 718–722.

Padgett, D. (2012). Writing a qualitative methods proposal for external funding. In *Qualitative and mixed methods in public health* (pp. 241–253). Thousand Oaks, CA: Sage.

Penrod, J. (2003). Getting funded: Writing a successful qualitative small-project proposal. *Qualitative Health Research*, 13, 821–832

Ritchie, J., & Lewis, J. (2003). Generalizing from qualitative research. In *Qualitative research practice: A guide for social science students and researchers* (pp. 263–286). London: Sage Publications.

Silverman D. (2011a). *Interpreting qualitative data* (4th ed.). London: Sage.

Assessing Qualitative Research

Barbour, R. (2001). Checklists for improving rigor in qualitative research: A case of the tail wagging the dog? *British Medical Journal*, 322, 1115–1117.

Guest, G., MacQueen, K., & Namey, E. (2012). Validity and reliability (credibility and dependability) in qualitative research and data analysis. In *Applied thematic analysis* (pp. 79–106). Thousand Oaks, CA: Sage.

Malterud, K. (2001). Qualitative research: Standards, challenges and guidelines. Lancet, 358(9280), 483–488.

Morse, J. (2003) A review committee's guide for evaluating qualitative proposals. *Qualitative Health Research*, 13, 833–851.

Ritchie, J., & Lewis, J. (2003). Generalising from qualitative research. In *Qualitative research practice: A guide for social science students and researchers* (pp. 263–286). London: Sage Publications.

Silverman D. (2011a). Credible qualitative research. In *Interpreting qualitative data* (4th ed.) (pp. 351–393). London: Sage.

REFERENCES

Atherton, M., Bellis-Smith, N., Chichero, J., & Suter, M. (2007). Texture-modified foods and thickened fluids as used for individuals with dysphagia: Australian standardised labels and definitions. *Nutrition and Dietetics*, 64, S53–S76.

Barbour, R. (2001). Checklists for improving rigor in qualitative research: A case of the tail wagging the dog? *British Medical Journal*, 322(7294), 115–117.

Barbour, R. (2007). *Doing focus groups. The SAGE Qualitative Research Kit.* London: Sage Publications.

Belgrave, L., Zablotsky, D., & Guadagno, M. (2002). How do we talk to each other? Writing qualitative research for quantitative readers. *Qualitative Health Research*, 12(10), 1427–1439.

Berg, B. (2007). A dramaturgical look at interviewing. In *Qualitative research methods for the social sciences* (6th ed., pp. 89–143). Boston, MA: Allyn & Bacon.

Bernard, H., & Ryan, G. (2010). *Analyzing qualitative data: Systematic approaches.* Thousand Oaks, CA: Sage Publications.

Bloor, M., Frankland, J., Thomas, M., & Robson, K. (2001). *Focus groups in social research.* London: Sage Publications.

Bluff, R. (1997). Evaluating qualitative research. *British Journal of Midwifery*, 5(4), 232–235.

Bogdan, R., & Taylor, S. (1975). *Introduction to qualitative research methods.* New York: John Wiley and Sons.

Brondani, M., MacEntee, M., Bryant, S., & O'Neill, B. (2008). Using written vignettes in focus groups among older adults to discuss oral health as a sensitive topic. *Qualitative Health Research*, 18(8), 1145–1153.

Carey, M. (1995). Issues and applications of focus groups: Introduction. *Qualitative Health Research*, 5(4), 413.

Charmaz, K. (2006). *Constructing grounded theory: A practical guide through qualitative analysis.* London: Sage Publications.

Colucci, E. (2007). Focus groups can be fun: The use of activity oriented questions in focus group discussions. *Qualitative Health Research*, 17(10), 1422–1433.

Conradson, D. (2005). Focus groups. In R. Flowerdew & D. Martin (Eds.). *Methods in human geography: A guide for students doing a research project* (pp. 128–143). Harlow, UK: Pearson Prentice Hall.

Contino, R. (2012). *Perceptions of diabetes, hypertension, healthy eating, and physical activity within the Bhutanese refugee community living in metro Atlanta* (Unpublished master's thesis). Emory University, Atlanta, GA.

Cooper, C., Jorgensen, C., & Merritt, T. (2003). Telephone focus groups: An emerging method in public health research. *Journal of Women's Health, 12*(10), 945–951.

Cooper, C., Saraiya, M., McLean, T., Hannan, J., Liesmann, J., Rose, S., & Lawson, H. (2005). Pap test intervals used by physicians serving low income women through the National Breast and Cervical cancer Early Detection Program. *Journal of Women's Health, 14*, 670–678.

Cooper, C., & Yarbrough, S. (2010). Tell me-show me: Using combined focus group and photovoice methods to gain understanding of health issues in rural Guatemala. *Qualitative Health Research, 20*(5), 644–653.

Corbin, J., & Strauss, A. (2008). Basics of qualitative research: Grounded theory procedures and techniques (3rd ed.). Thousand Oaks, CA: Sage.

Corden, A., & Sainsbury, R. (1996, July). *Using quotations in qualitative research.* Paper presented to the Fourth International Social Science Methodology Conference, University of Essex, United Kingdom.

Daley, C., James, A., Ulrey, E., Joseph, S., Talawyma, A., Choi, W., Greiner, K., Coe, M. (2010). Using focus groups in community-based participatory research: Challenges and resolutions. *Qualitative Health Research, 20*(5), 697–706.

David, M., & Sutton, C. (2004). *Social research: The basics.* London: Sage Publications.

Denzin, N. (1989). *The research act* (3rd ed.). Englewood Cliffs, NJ: Prentice Hall.

Denzin, N., & Lincoln, Y. (2000). The discipline and practice of qualitative research. In N. Denzin & Y. Lincoln (Eds.), *Handbook of qualitative research* (2nd ed.) (pp. 1–47). Thousand Oaks, CA: Sage Publications.

Denzin, N., & Lincoln, Y. (Eds.). (2008). *Collecting and interpreting qualitative materials* (3rd ed.). Thousand Oaks, CA: Sage Publications.

Diamond, I., Stephenson, R., Sheppard, Z., Smith, A., Hayward, S., Heatherley, S., & Stansfeld, S. (2000). *Perceptions of aircraft noise, sleep and health.* United Kingdom: Civil Aviation Authority.

Dixon-Woods, R., Shaw, L., Agarwal, S., & Smith, J. (2004). The problem of appraising qualitative research. *Quality Safety Health Care, 13*, 223–225.

Duggleby, W. (2005). What about focus group interaction data? *Qualitative Health Research, 15*(6), 832–840.

Easton, K., McComish, J., & Greenberg, R. (2000). Avoiding common pitfalls in qualitative data collection and transcription. *Qualitative Health Research, 10*(5), 703–707.

Elliott, J. (2005). *Using narrative in social research: Qualitative and quantitative approaches.* London: Sage Publications.

Fern, E. (1982). The use of focus groups for idea generation: The effects of group size, acquaintanceship, and moderator on response quality and quality. *Journal of Marketing Research, 19*, 1–13.

Fern, E. (2001). *Advanced focus group research.* Thousand Oaks, CA: Sage Publications.

Fielding, N. (Ed.). (1988). *Actions and structure.* London: Sage Publications.

Finlay, L. (2002). Outing the researcher: The provenance, process and practice of reflexivity. *Qualitative Health Research, 12*(4), 531–545.

Finaly, L., & Gough, B. (2003). *Reflexivity: A practical guide for researchers in health and social sciences.* Oxford: Blackwell.

Flick, U. (2002). *An introduction to qualitative research* (2nd ed.). London: Sage Publications.

Flick, U. (2007). *Managing quality in qualitative research. The SAGE Qualitative Research Kit.* London: Sage Publications.

Flick, U. (2009). *An introduction to qualitative research* (4th ed.). London: Sage Publications.

Fox, F., Morris, M., & Rumsey, N. (2007). Doing synchronous online focus groups with young people: Methodological reflections. *Qualitative Health Research, 17*(4), 539–547.

Giacomini, G., & Cook, D. (2000). Users guide to the medical literature XXII: Qualitative research in healthcare. Are results of the study valid? *JAMA, 284,* 357–362.

Gibson, F. (2007). Conducting focus groups with children and young people: Strategies for success. *Journal of Research in Nursing, 12*(45), 473–483.

Glaser, B., & Strauss, A. (1967). *The discovery of grounded theory: Strategies for qualitative research.* New York: Aldine de Gruyter.

Grace, C., Begum, R., Subhani, S., Kopelman, P., & Greenhalgh, T. (2008). Prevention of type 2 diabetes in British Bangladeshis: Qualitative study of community, religious and professional perspectives. *British Medical Journal Online First, 337,* a1931

Grbich, C. (2007). *Qualitative data analysis: An introduction.* London: Sage Publications.

Green, J., & Thorogood, N. (2004). *Qualitative methods for health research.* London: Sage Publications.

Green, J., & Thorogood, N. (2009). *Qualitative methods for health research* (2nd ed.). London: Sage Publications.

Greenbaum, T. (2000). *Moderating focus groups. A practical guide for group facilitation.* Thousand Oaks, CA: Sage Publications.

Guest, G., MacQueen, K., & Namey, E. (2012). *Applied thematic analysis.* Thousand Oaks, CA: Sage.

Hammersley, M. (1990). *Reading ethnographic research: A critical guide.* London: Longman.

Hammersley, M. (1992). *What's wrong with ethnography?* London: Routledge.

Hennink, M. (2007). *International focus group research: A handbook for the health and social sciences.* Cambridge: Cambridge University Press.

Hennink, M. (2008). Language and communication in cross-cultural qualitative research. In P. Liamputtong (Ed.), Doing cross cultural research: Ethical and methodological perspectives (pp. 21–34). Netherlands: Springer Publishers.

Hennink, M., & Diamond, I. (1999). Using focus groups in social research. In A. Memnon & R. Bull (Eds.), *Handbook of the psychology of interviewing* (pp. 113–141). Chichester, UK: John Wiley and Sons Ltd.

Hennink, M., Hutter, I., & Bailey, A. (2011). *Qualitative research methods.* London: Sage Publications.

Hennink, M., & McFarland, D. (2013). A delicate web: Household changes in health behaviour enabled by microcredit in Burkina Faso. *Global Public Health*, 8(2), 144–158.

Hennink, M., & Madise, N. (2005). Influence of user fees for reproductive health in Malawi. *African Population Studies*, 20(2), 125–141.

Hennink, M., Rana, I., & Iqbal, R. (2005). Knowledge of personal and sexual development amongst young people in Pakistan. *Culture, Health and Sexuality*, 7(4), 319–332.

Hennink, M., & Weber, M. (2013). Quality issues of court reporters and transcriptionists for qualitative research. *Qualitative Health Research*, 23(5), 700–710.

Hesse-Biber, S., & Leavy, P. (2006). *The practice of qualitative research.* Thousand Oaks, CA: Sage Publications.

Holmes, K., Winskell, K., Hennink, M., & Chidiac, S. (2011). Microfinance and HIV mitigation among people living with HIV in the era of anti-retroviral therapy: Emerging lessons from Cote d'Ivoire. *Global Public Health*, 6, 447–461.

Hopkins, P. (2007). Thinking critically and creatively about focus groups. *Area*, 39(4), 528–535.

Huffman, S., Veen, J., Hennink, M., & McFarland, D. (2012). Exploitation, vulnerability to tuberculosis and access to treatment among Uzbek labor migrants in Kazakhstan. *Social Science and Medicine*, 74, 864–872.

Humbert, M., Chad, K., Spink, K., Muhajarine, N., Anderson, K., Bruner, M., Girolami, T., Odnokon, P., Gryba, C. (2006). Factors that influence physical activity participation among high- and low-SES youth. *Qualitative Health Research*, 16(4), 467–483.

Hurworth, R. (2004). Telephone focus groups. *Social Research Update*, 44. Retrieved from http://sru.soc.surrey.ac.uk/SRU44.html

International HIV/AIDS Alliance. (2006). *Tools together now! 100 participatory tools to mobilize communities for HIV/AIDS.* Retrieved from http://www.aidsalliance.org/includes/Publication/Tools_Together_Now_2009.pdf

Jennings, B., Loan, L., Heiner, S., Hemman, E., & Swanson, K. (2005). Soldiers' experiences with military health care. *Military Medicine*, 170(12), 999–1004.

Jette, S., Wilson, B., & Sparks, R. (2007). Female youths' perceptions of smoking in popular films. *Qualitative Health Research*, 17(3), 323–339.

Kick, S., Adams, L., & O'Brien-Gonzales, A. (2000). Unique issues of older medical students. *Teaching and Learning in Medicine*, 12(3), 150–155.

Kirk, J., & Miller, M. (1986). *Reliability and validity in qualitative research.* Qualitative Research Methods Series: Vol. 1. London: Sage Publications.

Kitzinger, J. (1994). The methodology of focus groups: The importance of interaction between research participants. *Sociology of Health and Illness*, 16, 103–121.

Kitzinger, J. (2005). Focus group research: Using group dynamics to explore perceptions, experiences and understandings. In I. Holloway (Ed.), *Qualitative research in healthcare* (pp. 56–70). Maidenhead, UK: Open University Press.

Kitzinger, J., & Barbour, R. (1999). Introduction: The challenge and promise of focus groups. In R. Barbour & J. Kitzinger (Eds.), *Developing focus group research: Politics, theory and practice* (pp. 1–20). London: Sage Publications.

Knodel, J. (1995). Focus group research on the living arrangements of elderly in Asia [Special issue]. *Journal of Cross Cultural Gerontology*, 10, 1–162.

Knodel, J., Chamratrithirong, A., Debavala, N. (1987). *Thailand's reproductive revolution: Rapid fertility decline in a third world setting*. Madison, WI: University of Wisconsin Press.

Knodel, J., Havanon, N., & Pramualratana, A. (1984). Fertility transition in Thailand: A qualitative analysis. *Population and development review*, 10(2), 297–315.

Koppelman, N., & Bourjolly, J. (2001). Conducting focus groups with women with severe psychiatric disabilities: A methodological overview. *Psychiatric Rehabilitation Journal*, 25(2), 142–151.

Krippendorf, K. (2004). *Content analysis: An introduction to its methodology* (2nd ed.). Thousand Oaks, CA: Sage.

Kroll, T., Barbour, R., & Harris, J. (2007). Using focus groups in disability research. *Qualitative Health Research*, 17(5), 690–698.

Krueger, R. (1988). *Practical guide for applied research*. Thousand Oaks, CA: Sage Publications.

Krueger, R. (1998). *Developing questions for focus groups. Focus Group Kit 3*. Thousand Oaks, CA: Sage Publications.

Krueger, R., & Casey, M. (2000). *Focus groups: A practical guide for applied research* (3rd ed.). Thousand Oaks, CA: Sage Publications.

Krueger, R., & Casey, M. (2009). *Focus groups: A practical guide for applied research* (4th ed.). Thousand Oaks, CA: Sage Publications.

Lam, W., Fielding, R., Johnson, J., Tin, K., & Leung, G. (2004). Identifying barriers to the adoption of evidence-based medicine practice in clinical clerks: A longitudinal focus group study. *Medial Education*, 38, 987–997.

Liamputtong, P. (2011). *Focus group methodology*. London: Sage Publications.

Liamputtong, P., & Ezzy, D. (2007). *Qualitative research methods* (2nd ed.). Melbourne, Australia: Oxford University Press.

Lincoln, Y., & Guba, E. (1985). *Naturalistic inquiry*. Beverley Hills, CA: Sage Publications.

Lynch, M. (2000). Against reflexivity as an academic virtue and source of privileged knowledge. *Theory, Culture and Society*, 17(3), 26–54

MacPhail, C., Sayles, J., Cummingham, W., & Newman, P. (2012). Perceptions of sexual risk compensation following post trial HIV vaccine uptake among young South Africans. *Qualitative Health Research*, 22(5), 668–678.

Madriz, E. (2003). Focus groups in feminist research. In N. K. Denzin & Y. S. Lincoln (Eds.), *Collecting and interpreting qualitative materials* (2nd ed., pp. 363–388). Thousand Oaks, CA: Sage.

Mason, J. (1996). *Qualitative researching*. London: Sage Publications.

Mason, J. (2002). *Qualitative researching* (2nd ed.). London: Sage Publications.

Maynard-Tucker, G. (2000). Conducting focus groups in developing countries: Skill training for bi-lingual facilitators. *Qualitative Health Research*, 10(3), 396–410.

Mays, N., & Pope, C. (2000). Assessing quality in qualitative research. *British Medical Journal*, 320, 50–52.

Merton, R. (1987). The focused interview and focus groups. Continuities and discontinuities. *Public Opinion Quarterly*, 51, 550–566.

Merton, R., & Kendall, P. (1946). The focused interview. *American Journal of Sociology*, 51, 541–557.

Mkandawire-Valhmu, L., & Stevens, P. (2010). The critical value of focus group discussions in research with women living with HIV in Malawi. *Qualitative Health Research*, 20(5), 684–696.

Moisander, J., & Valtonen, A. (2006). *Qualitative marketing research: A cultural approach*. Introducing Qualitative Methods Series. London: Sage Publications.

Morgan, D. (Ed.). (1993). *Successful focus groups. Advancing the state of the art*. Newbury Park, CA: Sage Publications.

Morgan, D. (1997). *Focus groups as qualitative research* (2nd ed.). Qualitative Research Methods Series: Vol. 16. Thousand Oaks, CA: Sage Publications.

Morgan, D. (2010). Reconsidering the role of interaction in analysing and reporting focus groups. *Qualitative Health Research*, 20(5), 718–722.

Morgan, D., & Krueger, R. (1993). When to use focus groups and why. In D. Morgan (Ed.), *Successful focus groups: Advancing the state of the art* (pp. 3–19). Newbury Park, CA: Sage Publications.

Morse, J., Barrett, M., Mayan, M., Olson, K., & Spiers, J. (2002). Verification strategies for establishing reliability and validity in qualitative research. *International Journal of Qualitative Methods*, 1(2), 1–19.

Mturi, A., & Hennink, M. (2005). Perceptions of sex education for adolescents in Lesotho. *Culture Health and Sexuality*, 7(2), 129–143.

Munday, J. (2006). Identity in focus: The use of focus groups to study the construction of collective identity. *Sociology*, 40(1), 89–105.

National Commission for the Protection of Human Subjects of Behavioral Research. (1978). *The Belmont Report: Ethical principles and guidelines for the protection of human subjects of research* (DHEW Publication No. OS 78-0012). Washington DC: Department of Health, Education, and Welfare.

Newhouse, R. P. (2005). Exploring nursing issues in rural hospitals. *Journal of Nursing Administration*, 35(7–8), 350–358.

O'Donnell, A., Lutfey, K., Marceau, L., & McKinlay, J. (2007). Using focus groups to improve the validity of cross-national survey research: A study of physician decision-making. *Qualitative Health Research*, 17(7), 971–981.

Owen, S. (2001). The practical, methodological and ethical dilemmas of conducting focus groups with vulnerable clients. *Journal of Advanced Nursing*, 36(5), 652–658.

Padgett, D. (2012). Qualitative and mixed methods in public health. Thousand Oaks, CA: Sage Publications.

Parker, A., & Tritter, J. (2006). Focus group method and methodology: Current practice and recent debate. *International Journal of Research and Method in Education*, 29(1), 23–37.

Patenaude, A. (2004). No promises, but I'm willing to listen and tell what I hear: Conducting qualitative research among prison inmates and staff. *The Prison Journal*, 84, 69S–91S.

Patton, M. (1990). *Qualitative evaluation and research methods* (2nd ed.). Newbury Park, CA: Sage Publications.

Phillips, N., & Hardy, C. (2002). *Discourse analysis: Investigating processes of social construction*. Qualitative Research Methods Series, Vol. 50. Thousand Oaks, CA: Sage Publications.

Pillow, W. (2003). Confession, catharsis or cure? Rethinking the issues of reflexivity as methodological power in qualitative research. *International Journal of Qualitative Studies in Education*, 16(2), 175–96.

Pollack, S. (2003). Focus-group methodology in research with incarcerated women: Race, power, and collective experience. *Affilia*, 18, 461–472.

Quintiliani, L., Campbell, M., Haines, P., & Weber, K. (2008). The use of the pile sort method in identifying groups of healthful lifestyle behaviors among female community college students. *Journal of the American Dietetic Association*, 108, 1503–1507.

Ragnarsson, A., Onya, H., Thorson, A., Ekstrom, A., & Aaro, L. (2008). Young males' gendered sexuality in the era of HIV and AIDS in Limpopo Province, South Africa. *Qualitative Health Research*, 18(6), 739–746.

Rapley, T. (2007). *Doing conversation, discourse and document analysis. The SAGE Qualitative Research Kit*. London: Sage Publications.

Rapley, T. (2011). Some pragmatics of qualitative data analysis. In D. Silverman (Ed.), *Qualitative research* (3rd ed., pp. 273–290). London: Sage.

Ritchie, J., & Lewis, J. (2003). *Qualitative research practice: A guide for social science students and researchers*. London: Sage Publications.

Ross, L., Stroud, L., Rose, S., & Jorgensen, C. (2006). Using telephone focus group methodology to examine prostate cancer screening practices of African-American primary care physicians. *Journal of the National Medical Association*, 98, 1296–1299.

Rubin, H., & Rubin, I. (2005). *Qualitative interviewing: The art of hearing data* (2nd ed.). Thousand Oaks, CA: Sage Publications.

Scott, S., Sharpe, H., O'Leary, K., Dehaeck, U., Hindmarsh, K., Moore, J. G., & Osmond, M. (2009). Court reporters: A viable solution for the challenges of focus group data collection? *Qualitative Health Research*, 19(1), 140–146.

Seale, C. (1999). *The quality of qualitative research*. Introducing Qualitative Methods Series. London: Sage Publications.

Sheu, J., Ephraim, P., Powe, N., Rabb, H., Senga, M., Evans, K., Joor, B., Crews, D., Grer, R., Boulware, E. (2012). African American and non-African American patients' and families decision making about renal replacement therapies. *Qualitative Health Research*, 22(7), 997–1006.

Silverman D. (2011a). *Interpreting qualitative data* (4th ed.). London: Sage.

Silverman D. (Ed.). (2011b). *Qualitative research: Issues of theory, methods and practice* (3rd ed.). London: Sage.

Smith, J., Sullivan, S., & Baxter, G. (2009). Telephone focus groups in physiotherapy research: Potential uses and recommendations. *Physiotherapy Theory and Practice*, 25(4), 241–256.

Smithson, J. (2008). Focus groups. In P. Alasuutari, L. Bickman, & J. Brannen (Eds.), *The Sage handbook of social research methods* (pp. 357–430). London; Sage.

Stewart, D., & Shamdasani, R. (1990). *Focus groups: Theory and practice.* Applied Social Research Methods Series, Vol. 20. Newbury Park, CA: Sage Publications.

Stewart, D., Shamdasani, R., & Rook, D. (2007). *Focus groups: Theory and practice* (2nd ed.). Thousand Oaks, CA: Sage.

Strauss, A., & Corbin, J. (1998). *Basics of qualitative research: Techniques and procedures for developing grounded theory* (2nd ed.). Thousand Oaks, CA: Sage Publications

Tashakkori, A., & Teddlie, C. (1998). *Mixed methodology: Combining qualitative and quantitative approaches.* Thousand Oaks, CA: Sage Publications.

Ulin, P., Robinson, E., & Tolley, E. (2005). *Qualitative methods in public health: A field guide for applied research.* San Francisco, CA: Jossey Bass.

Ulin, P., Robinson, E., Tolley, E., & McNeill, E. (2002). *Qualitative methods: A field guide for applied research in sexual and reproductive health.* Research Triangle Park, NC: Family Health International.

Vaughn, S., Shay Schumm, J., & Sinagub, J. (1996). *Focus group interviews in education and psychology.* Thousand Oaks, CA: Sage Publications.

Weber, R. (1990). *Basic content analysis* (2nd ed.). Newbury Park, CA: Sage.

Wilkinson, S. (1998). Focus groups in health research: Exploring the meaning of health and illness. *Journal of Health Psychology, 3*(3), 329–348.

Wilkinson, S. (2004). Focus groups: A feminist method. In S. Hesse-Biber & M. Yaiser (Eds.), *Feminist perspectives on social research* (pp. 271–295). New York: Oxford University Press.

Wilkinson, S. (2011). Analysing focus group data. In D. Silverman (Ed.), *Qualitative research* (3rd ed., pp. 168–186). London: Sage

Wolcott, H. (2001). *Writing up qualitative research* (2nd ed.). Thousand Oaks, CA: Sage Publications.

Wong, Y., Sands, R., & Solomon, P. (2010). Conceptualizing community: The experience of mental health consumers. *Qualitative Health Research, 20*(5), 654–667.

Woods-Giscombe, C. (2010). Superwoman schema: African American women's views on stress, strength and health. *Qualitative Health Research, 20*(5), 668–683.

World Medical Association (WMA) (2008). World Medical Association Declaration of Helsinki, Ethical Principles of Medical research involving Human subjects. Retrieved from http://www.wma.net/en/30publications/10policies/b3/index.html

ABOUT THE AUTHOR

Monique M. Hennink is Associate Professor of Global Health at the Rollins School of Public Health, Emory University. Trained in social geography and demography in Australia, she was based in the United Kingdom for 14 years conducting reproductive health research mostly in developing countries, and for the past decade has focused on public health research more broadly. Her research focuses on examining the social, cultural, and contextual influences on human behavior and promoting behavior change. Her research topics include microcredit, health, and women's empowerment; sexual and reproductive health; childhood obesity and diabetes; and safe water, sanitation, and hygiene. She has extensive experience in applying qualitative research in developing country settings and among minority populations. She teaches graduate courses in qualitative research methods at Emory University and leads research training workshops worldwide. She is author of *International Focus Group Discussions* (Cambridge University Press, 2007) and coauthor of *Qualitative Research Methods* (Sage Publications, 2011).

INDEX